THE GLUTEN-FREE
SLOW  COOKER

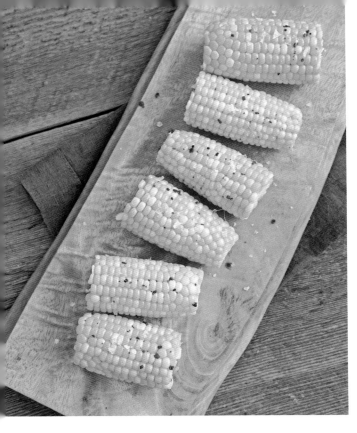
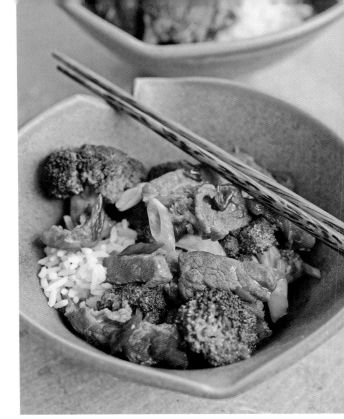
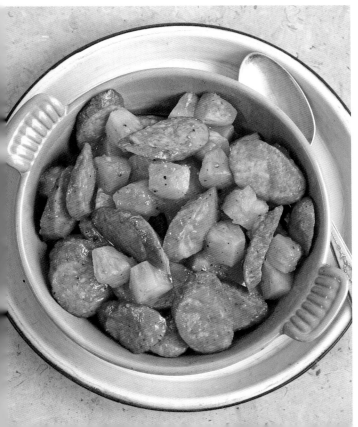
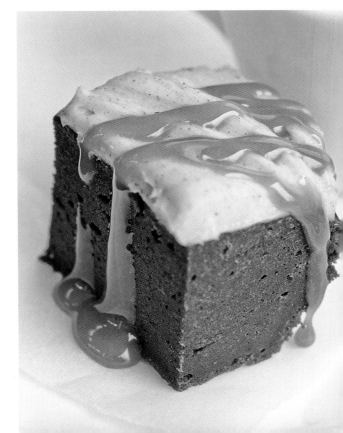

THE GLUTEN-FREE
SLOW COOKER

Set It and Go with Quick and Easy Wheat-Free Meals Your Whole Family Will Love

HOPE COMERFORD

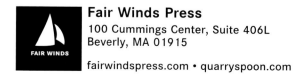

Fair Winds Press
100 Cummings Center, Suite 406L
Beverly, MA 01915

fairwindspress.com • quarryspoon.com

© 2015 Fair Winds Press
Text © 2015 Hope Comerford

First published in the USA in 2015 by
Fair Winds Press, a member of
Quarto Publishing Group USA Inc.
100 Cummings Center
Suite 406-L
Beverly, MA 01915-6101
www.fairwindspress.com

Visit www.QuarrySPOON.com and help us celebrate food and
culture one spoonful at a time!

19 18 17 16 15   1 2 3 4 5

ISBN: 978-1-59233-697-5

Digital edition published in 2015
eISBN: 978-1-62788-756-4

Library of Congress Cataloging-in-Publication Data
Comerford, Hope.
  The gluten-free slow cooker : set it and go with quick and easy
  wheat-free meals your whole family will love / Hope Comerford.
    pages cm
  ISBN 978-1-59233-697-5 (paperback)
1. Gluten-free diet--Recipes. 2. Gluten-free foods. 3. Electric
cooking, Slow. I. Title.
  RM237.86.C65 2015
  641.5'638--dc23   2015005603

Cover and book design by Georgia Rucker
Book layout by *tabula rasa* graphic design
Photography by JNV
Food & Prop Styling by Ross Yedinak

Printed and bound in China

The information in this book is for educational purposes
only. It is not intended to replace the advice of a physician or
medical practitioner. Please see your health care provider before
beginning any new health program.

To my incredibly supportive husband, Justin,
my daughter, Ella and my son, Gavin: You inspire me
to cook every day. Without your constant support
and encouragement, this book would not have
been possible. I love you, my beautiful family!

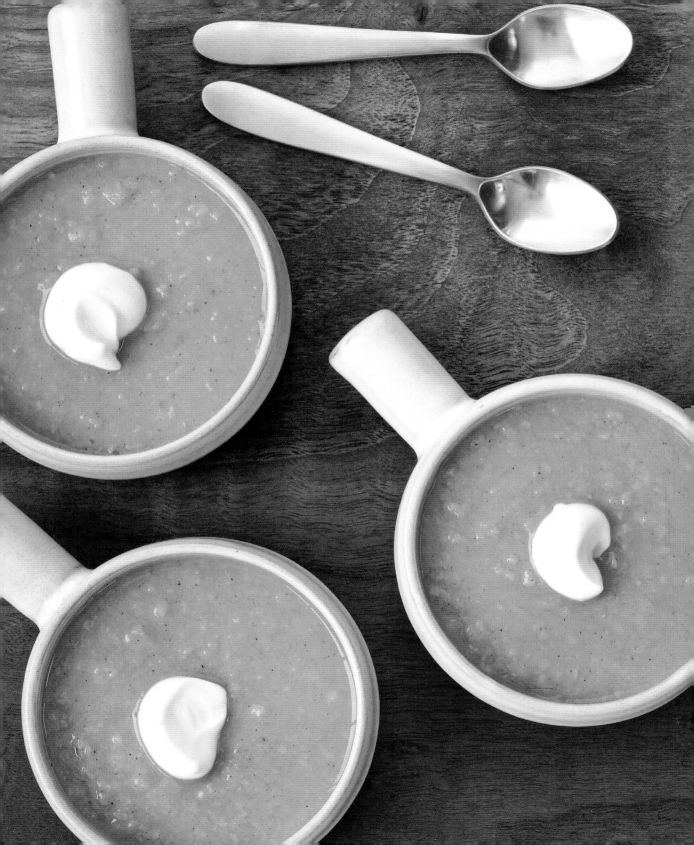

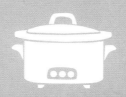

CONTENTS

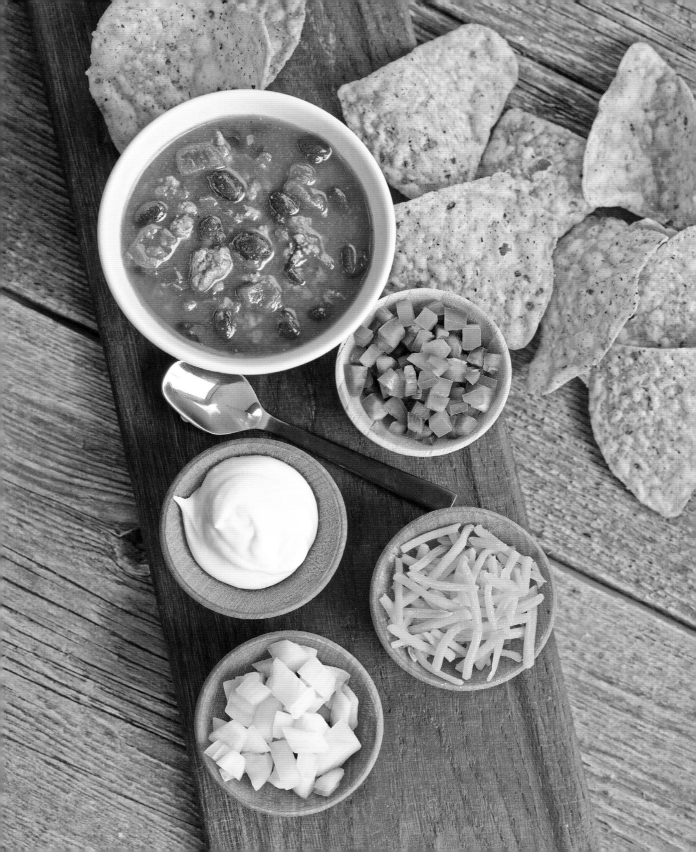

CHAPTER 1

THE BASICS OF GLUTEN-FREE SLOW COOKING

As busy as life is, throwing gluten-free cooking into the mix can feel like a huge and daunting task. Fear not! You're holding in your hand more than 100 delicious, gluten-free recipes you can make quickly and easily in your slow cooker—recipes your entire family will love, gluten-free or not. So, whether your whole family is gluten-free, or it's just you, your spouse, your daughter, or some other relative or friend, you've come to the right place!

MY STORY

In 2013, I was diagnosed as being gluten-intolerant. After I had suffered for twenty years with severe stomach pains, I was put through every test my doctors could think of. Until my diagnosis, I had no idea gluten was the problem. Once I cut it out, I was amazed at how good I felt. I didn't have to suffer every day of my life!

That said, being gluten-free can also bring its own challenges. I'm no longer able to fly through a drive-through and grab a quick bite to eat. I can't go to a family gathering without questioning *everything* that's set out to eat. Most of the time, I try to bring a dish or two to share that I know I can have and will fill me up. That's where these recipes come in. You can throw one or two of them in your slow cooker and bring a delicious and healthy dish to any gathering you go to—even if that gathering is at your own kitchen table.

I began my blog, A Busy Mom's Slow Cooker Adventures, in 2010 to share my slow cooker recipes with my family and coworkers. It morphed into a *gluten-free* slow cooker blog three years later, following my diagnosis. Due to my new lifestyle, I naturally began to cook healthier, and I haven't looked back since. I'm a wife to my wonderful husband of nine years, and we have two beautiful children, ages seven and four. Though they aren't gluten-free, we all love eating meals that are, and we hope that you will too.

Before we get into the recipes though, let's get some basics out of the way first.

Choosing a Slow Cooker: What Size Do I Need?

I'm frequently asked about how to choose a slow cooker, and my answer is that it really isn't hard at all. To choose the correct size for your family, follow this guideline:

USE	SLOW COOKER SIZE
Dips and sauces	1 quart (1 L) or small warmer
Appetizers	2 to 3 quart (2 to 3 L)
2 to 3 person household	3 to 5 quart (3.8 to 5 L)
4 to 5 person household	5 to 6 quart (5 to 6 L)
6+ person household	7 quart (6.6 L)

Programmable versus Manual Slow Cookers

With so many different types of slow cookers out there, which one will you choose? Read on to see which type of slow cooker best suits your needs.

PROGRAMMABLE SLOW COOKERS

If you are a person who is away from the house for long periods of time (longer than 6 to 8 hours), then a programmable slow cooker would be perfect for you. Programmable slow cookers will automatically switch over to the WARM setting when the set cook time is done. They have saved *many* meals for me. Because of the convenience of the technology, programmable slow cookers are more expensive than manual slow cookers. However, in my opinion, they are worth every penny.

MANUAL SLOW COOKERS

If you don't plan on being away from your slow cooker for longer than 6 to 8 hours, then a manual slow cooker should be just fine for you, because you'll be around to turn the slow cooker off or to warm manually. Manual slow cookers are much cheaper than programmable slow cookers, and they work great.

What Brand Slow Cooker Should I Buy?

Honestly, everyone has their opinion on which brand they feel is best. My best advice to you is to read reviews online of each slow cooker you're considering before making a purchase. Some slow cookers tend to cook "hotter" than others, making some people feel that their food cooks too fast. I hear this complaint a lot. If you ever have a concern with the way a slow cooker is cooking, contact the manufacturer. They may be able to offer you some advice on their product. I tend to stick with Crock-Pot Slow Cookers because I find they cook most consistently for me.

Slow Cooking Tips and Tricks

I've learned a lot of tips and tricks along my slow-cooking journey. I'm sharing some of my favorite with you so you don't have to go through the bumps and bruises I did when I first started slow-cooking.

Invest in some liners. You should know a secret. Wonderful things called *slow cooker liners*, which can be found near the aluminum foil at most grocery stores, act kind of like an oven bag for your slow cooker. They are absolutely wonderful because you put them in the crock, add your ingredients, cook, and then throw away the liner when you're done. They literally make for zero-cleanup cooking! They are also BPA free and approved by the FDA for cooking.

Spray with cooking spray. If you're not using a liner, spray the crock of your slow cooker with non-stick cooking spray each time you cook, especially when you're making anything with cheese or sugar in it. This will help you get the food out easier, and it will make cleanup a whole lot easier later. If you're having a very tough time removing something from your crock, try Bar Keepers Friend, which can be found near the household cleaning items in most stores. I've also heard filling your crock with hot water and letting it soak with a dryer sheet in it works well, too.

Fill appropriately. Slow cookers are intended to be filled one-half to three-quarters of the way full. Keep this in mind when choosing a slow cooker and when working with a particular recipe.

Understand your high and low. Ever wonder what the difference is between high and low? On low, the slow cooker reaches the simmer point at a slower rate than it does on high. When set on high, the slow cooker reaches the simmer point at a faster rate. So, when set on high, the slow cooker cooks the contents twice as fast. For instance, 4 hours on high is 8 hours on low, and vice versa.

Don't peek. Peeking is a no-no with slow cooking. Each time you lift that lid, you should add 20 more minutes to your cook time. So, unless a recipe calls for you to remove the lid or stir, don't do it. Resist the urge!

Plan accordingly. When planning your meals, think about the cook time for each of the recipes you want to make. Unless you have a programmable slow cooker that automatically switches to WARM when it's done cooking, if you know you're going to be away from the house longer than the recipe takes to cook, maybe save that one for another day. I tend to save my recipes with short cook times for days I'm either home from work or the weekends.

Try cheaper cuts of meat. Cheaper cuts of meat work great in the slow cooker because hours of slow cooking turn them into tender deliciousness.

Prep ahead. Some recipes/ingredients can be prepared in the crock the night before and refrigerated until the next morning for cooking. If you put the crock base in the refrigerator, always be sure to let it come back up to room temperature before turning it on, to prevent it from cracking.

Let it cool. When cleaning your crock, always let it cool before running water in it. Otherwise, you run the risk of cracking the crockery.

Mind your chicken cuts. Boneless skinless chicken breasts cook quickly in a slow cooker, and they cannot be cooked for the same amount of time as bone-in chicken. When substituting boneless skinless chicken for bone-in chicken in a recipe, you will need to reduce the cooking time.

The Gluten-Free Pantry

I want to give you a glimpse into my pantry because, as I said before, gluten-free cooking can be very overwhelming at first. The following are the common ingredients you'll find throughout this book. They are the ones I cook with on almost a daily basis. I don't use weird or hard-to-find ingredients. I am far too busy to be searching the grocery store for crazy things, and I don't have money to waste on ingredients that will only get used once.

FOOD ITEMS

Acorn squash
Allspice
Almonds, raw
Almond milk
Anaheim pepper
Apples
Arborio rice
Artichoke hearts
Avocado
Bacon
Baking soda
Bananas
Barbecue sauce, gluten-free
Basil, dried
Basil, fresh
Basil paste
Bay leaves
Beans, garbanzo (chickpeas)
Beans, kidney
Beans, navy
Beans, Northern, canned
Beef stock
Bell peppers
Bisquick, gluten-free
Black beans, canned
Black-eyed peas
Blueberries
Bread, gluten-free
Bread crumbs, gluten-free
Bread crumbs, panko, gluten-free

Broccoli, frozen
Brownie mix, gluten-free
Brown sugar
Butterscotch chips
Butter, unsalted
Cabbage
Cake mix, gluten-free, chocolate
Cake mix, gluten-free, yellow
Cannelloni beans
Carrots
Carrots, baby
Cashews, raw
Cauliflower, frozen
Cayenne pepper
Celery
Celery salt
Cereal, gluten-free, assorted
Cheese, Cheddar, shredded
Cheese, Colby jack, shredded
Cheese, Gouda
Cheese, Monterey jack
Cheese, mozzarella, balls, fresh
Cheese, mozzarella, shredded
Cheese, Parmesan, grated
Cheese, pepper jack
Cheese, sharp Cheddar, shredded
Cheese, Swiss, shredded
Chicken, bone-in
Chicken, boneless, skinless breasts
Chicken, boneless, skinless thighs
Chicken stock

Chicken, whole
Chicken wings
Chili powder
Chili sauce
Chipotles in adobo sauce
Chocolate chips, milk chocolate
Chocolate fudge pudding
Chocolate-hazelnut spread, such as Nutella
Chorizo, ground
Chuck roast
Cilantro
Cinnamon
Cloves, ground
Cocoa powder
Coconut oil
Condensed milk, sweetened
Coriander
Corn, frozen
Corn on the cob, frozen
Corn starch
Country Bob's all-purpose sauce
Cranberry sauce, whole berry
Cream cheese, reduced-fat
Cream, heavy
Cumin
Curry
Dates, pitted
Dried cranberries
Dry milk powder
Eggplant
Eggs
Egg whites
Enchilada sauce
English roast
Evaporated milk
Flank steak
Flour, gluten-free, such as Cup4Cup
Garam masala
Garlic
Garlic powder
Ginger powder
Green beans, fresh
Ground beef
Ground chicken
Ground sirloin

Ground turkey
Habanero pepper
Ham bone
Honey
Hot sauce
Instant coffee
Irish cream liqueur
Italian sausage, ground
Italian seasoning
Jalapeño pepper
Jalapeños, diced
Jalapeño, sliced in jar
Kahlua
Kielbasa, gluten-free
Kosher salt
Lamb, leg
Leeks
Lemon juice
Lentils
Lime juice
Limes
Mangos
Maple syrup
Marinara sauce
Milk
Minced garlic, fresh (in the jar)
Mrs. Dash Fiesta Lime Seasoning
Mrs. Dash Garlic and Herb Seasoning
Mrs. Dash Original Seasoning
Mrs. Dash Tomato Basil Garlic Seasoning
Mushrooms
Mushrooms, baby bella
Mustard powder, ground
Noodles, gluten-free lasagna
Nutmeg
Oats, old-fashioned
Oil, olive
Onion powder
Onions, green
Onions, red
Onions, white
Oranges
Oregano, dried
Paprika
Paprika, smoked

Parsley, dried
Parsley, fresh
Peaches
Peanut butter, natural, creamy
Pearl onions, frozen
Peas, frozen
Pecans, raw
Pepper, black, ground
Pineapple, chunks
Pistachios, raw
Pizza sauce
Poppy seed dressing
Pork chops
Pork loin, boneless
Pork roast, boneless
Pork shoulder roast
Potatoes
Potatoes, fingerling
Pretzels, gluten-free
Pumpkin pie spice
Pumpkin purée
Queso blanco
Quinoa
Raisins
Raisins, golden
Ranch dressing mix
Raspberries
Red pepper flakes
Rhubarb
Rice, brown
Rice, wild
Ricotta cheese
Rosemary, dried
Rosemary, fresh
Sage, dried
Sage, fresh
Salmon filets
Salsa
Salsa verde
Salt
Sausage, smoked
Sea salt
Sour cream
Southwest seasoning
Soy sauce, gluten-free

Spaghetti squash
Spinach, fresh
Spinach, frozen chopped
Sriracha
Steel cut oats
Stew meat
Strawberries, frozen
Sugar, granulated
Sugar, powdered
Sugar, turbinado
Sweet potatoes
Teriyaki sauce, gluten-free
Thyme, dried
Thyme, fresh
Tilapia filets
Tomatoes, diced
Tomatoes, crushed
Tomatoes, heirloom
Tomatoes, sun-dried
Tomato juice, no salt added
Tomato paste
Tomato sauce
Turkey breast
Turmeric
Vanilla
Vegetables, frozen mixed
Vegetables, frozen stir-fry
Vegetable shortening
Vegetable stock
Velveeta cheese
Vinegar, apple cider
Vinegar, rice
Walnuts, raw
Wine, white
Wing sauce
Worcestershire sauce
Yogurt, Greek, nonfat, plain

NONFOOD ITEMS
Aluminum foil
Butcher's twine
Mason jars, 6 ounces (175 ml)
Nonstick cooking spray
Parchment paper
Resealable bags

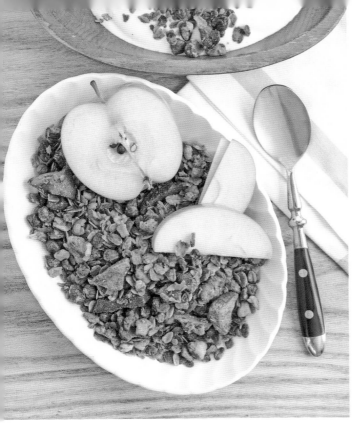
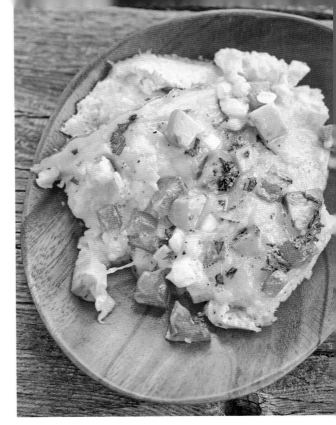
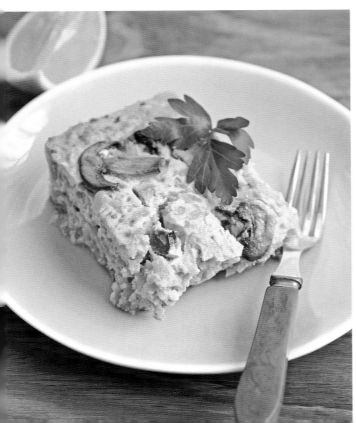
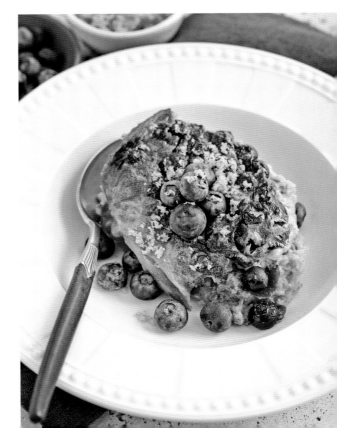

CHAPTER 2

WAKE UP TO BREAKFAST

Whether you're looking for a recipe that can cook all night or one that will cook up in a few hours, this chapter is full of tasty breakfast selections. From oatmeal to French toast, there's something for everyone.

Banana Pudding Breakfast Casserole

 DAIRY-FREE

Bread pudding for breakfast? Yup! Jazz up breakfast with a delicious and satisfying banana bread casserole, sprinkled with raisins and even more banana pieces. This is a sweet delight everyone will enjoy. Just be sure your bread cubes are nice and dry—the staler, the better!

10 eggs

2 cups (475 ml) almond milk

1 teaspoon vanilla

½ cup (100 g) turbinado sugar

1½ teaspoons cinnamon

¼ teaspoon nutmeg

1 loaf (8 x 5 inches, or 20 x 12.5 cm) gluten-free banana bread, cut into cubes and left out overnight to get stale

¼ cup (35 g) raisins

1½ cups (225 g) sliced banana

¼ cup (30 g) chopped walnuts (optional)

» Spray your crock with nonstick cooking spray.

» In a medium bowl, mix together the eggs, milk, vanilla, sugar, cinnamon, and nutmeg. Add the bread, raisins, bananas, and walnuts (if using) to this mixture and gently stir until everything is well coated. Pour the mixture into the crock.

» Cover the crock and cook on LOW for 4½ to 5 hours or on HIGH for 2 to 2½ hours.

RECOMMENDED SLOW COOKER SIZE:
3 to 4 quart (3 to 4 L)

YIELD: 8 servings

RECIPE NOTES

» **You can easily make this even healthier by swapping out the eggs for egg whites. If using packaged egg whites, just follow the measurements on the back of the carton to be the equivalent of ten eggs.**

» **To make clean-up an absolute cinch with this casserole, or any other that contains sugar, line your slow cooker with parchment paper or a slow cooker liner. It helps prevent hours of scrubbing and elbow grease.**

Banana Raspberry Oatmeal Casserole

 DAIRY-FREE

This delicious, lightly sweetened oatmeal casserole, glittered with pieces of banana and raspberries, is a healthy way to start your day, and it requires just a few simple ingredients.

2 bananas, sliced

2 cups (160 g) old-fashioned oats

⅓ cup (60 g) turbinado sugar

1 teaspoon baking soda

1 teaspoon cinnamon

¼ teaspoon salt

2 cups (475 ml) almond milk

2 tablespoons (25 g) coconut oil, melted

1 teaspoon vanilla

1 pint (455 g) raspberries

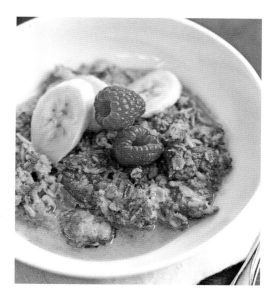

» Spray your crock with nonstick cooking spray, and then spread the bananas evenly around the bottom of the crock.

» In a bowl, mix together the oats, sugar, baking soda, cinnamon, and salt. Pour the mixture over the bananas.

» In a separate bowl, mix together the milk, oil, and vanilla. Spread the raspberries evenly over the top of oat mixture, and then pour the milk mixture over the top.

» Cover the crock and cook on LOW for 3½ to 4 hours or on HIGH for 2 hours.

RECOMMENDED SLOW COOKER SIZE:
5 to 6 quart (5 to 6 L)

YIELD: 4 to 6 servings

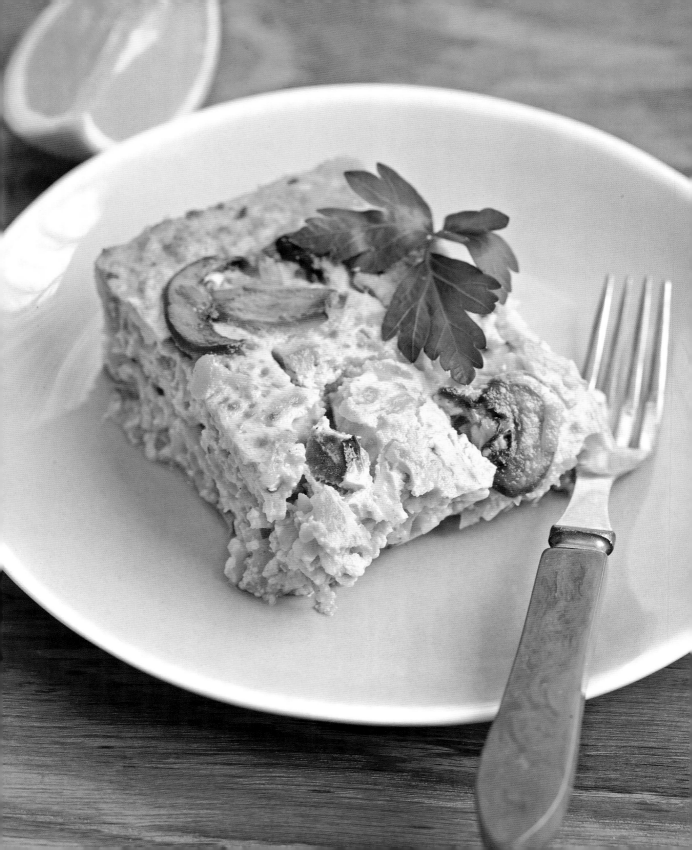

Cheesy Hash Brown Breakfast Casserole

Wake up in the morning to an entire delicious meal in one slow cooker. Hash browns, onions, mushrooms, ham, cheese, and eggs make this a complete, protein-packed breakfast.

6 eggs

1½ cups (350 g) nonfat plain Greek yogurt

½ cup (120 ml) chicken stock

1 teaspoon garlic powder

½ teaspoon salt

6 to 10 dashes hot sauce

½ cup (80 g) fresh minced onion

1 cup (110 g) shredded Swiss cheese

1 cup (120 g) shredded sharp Cheddar cheese

1 cup (150 g) diced cooked ham

1 cup (70 g) sliced mushrooms

2 pounds (900 g) frozen hash browns

» Spray your crock with nonstick cooking spray.

» In a large bowl, mix the eggs, yogurt, chicken stock, garlic powder, salt, and hot sauce. Stir in the onions, cheese, ham, and mushrooms.

» Add the hash browns and stir the mixture thoroughly. Dump the contents of the bowl into your crock.

» Cover the crock and cook on LOW for 7 to 9 hours or on HIGH for 3½ to 4½ hours.

RECOMMENDED SLOW COOKER SIZE:
5 quart (5 L) or larger

YIELD: 6 to 8 servings

 TIPS & SUGGESTIONS

Mix up your casserole by swapping the Swiss and sharp Cheddar cheese with two of your other favorite cheeses. You can also swap out the ham for cooked ground sausage, beef, or turkey. If you don't like mushrooms, use bell peppers, onions, or broccoli instead.

Fresh Frittata

Frittatas aren't just made on the stove top. This easy slow-cooker version is filled with tomatoes, avocados, and cilantro, making it fresh and healthy. It's a great way to start the day.

10 eggs

¼ cup grated (25 g) Parmesan cheese

8 dashes hot sauce

½ teaspoon salt

⅛ teaspoon ground black pepper

⅓ cup (55 g) chopped onion

½ cup (90 g) chopped tomato

½ cup (70 g) chopped avocado

¼ cup (4 g) chopped cilantro

» Spray your crock with nonstick cooking spray.

» In a bowl, mix together the eggs, cheese, hot sauce, salt, and pepper. Pour the mixture into your crock.

» Sprinkle the onion, tomato, avocado, and cilantro evenly over the egg mixture.

» Cover the crock and cook on LOW for 4 hours or on HIGH for 2 hours, or until the center is set.

RECOMMENDED SLOW COOKER SIZE:
3 to 5 quart (3 to 5 L)

YIELD: 4 to 6 servings

RECIPE NOTE

Using a fresh herb in this frittata makes all the difference. So, whether you use cilantro, or another herb in its place, use fresh! It's worth it.

TIPS & SUGGESTIONS

You can pack your fritatta with as many fresh veggies as you would like. The possibilities are endless. You can also add in meat, if you choose. Be creative and throw in whatever pleases the crowd you're serving!

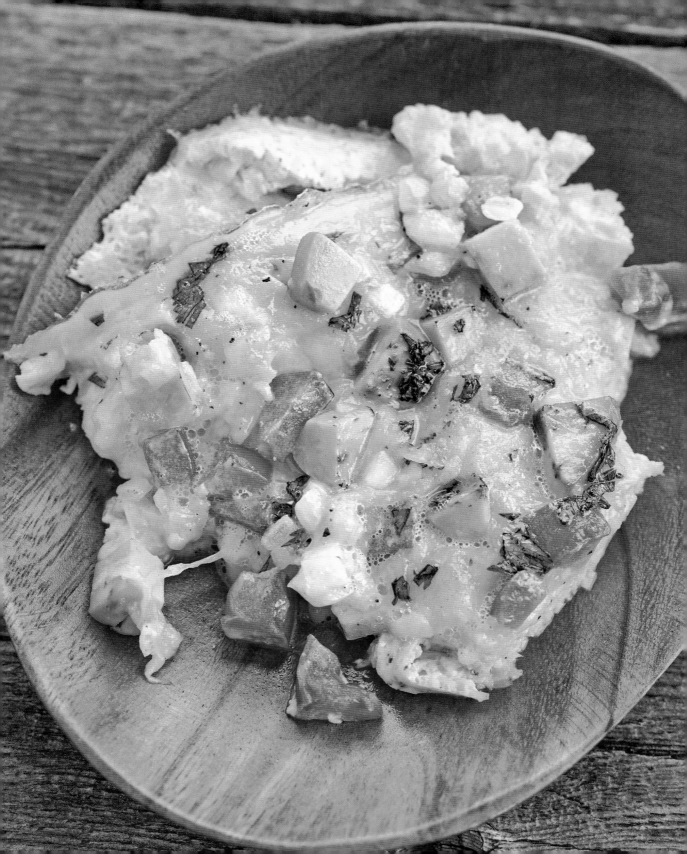

Peaches and Cream French Toast

Instead of slaving over the stove making French toast piece by piece, try this easy and incredibly flavorful casserole. If you love peaches and cream and French toast, you're going to *love* this tasty combo.

8 ounces (225 g) gluten-free bread, stale

1½ cups (355 ml) egg whites

1 cup (235 ml) almond milk

1 cup (235 ml) heavy cream

½ cup (115 g) brown sugar

2 tablespoons (12 g) orange zest

2 teaspoons (5 g) cinnamon

2 teaspoons (10 ml) vanilla

1 jar (24 ounces, or 680 g) peaches in
   light syrup, drained

» Spray your crock with nonstick cooking spray, and then place the bread inside.

» In a bowl, mix together the egg whites, milk, cream, sugar, orange zest, cinnamon, and vanilla.

» Spread the peaches over and around the bread. Pour the egg white mixture over the bread and peaches.

» Cover the crock and cook on LOW for 7 to 8 hours or on HIGH for 3½ to 4 hours.

RECOMMENDED SLOW COOKER SIZE:
3 to 4 quart (3 to 4 L)

YIELD: 4 to 6 servings

 RECIPE NOTE

» I have to tell you ... this isn't the prettiest casserole when it's done. For some reason, gluten-free bread tends to turn a brownish color after cooking. The taste of this, however, is phenomenal and it will make up for any lack in appearance. Put some whipped cream on top, and no one will notice.

Southern-Style Potato Bake

As a side dish, or as a main dish, this flavorful bake will make you want to come back for seconds. This easy-to-throw-together dish contains Southern potatoes mixed with turkey sausage and a creamy cheese sauce. What's not to love about that?

32 ounces (900 g) frozen diced potatoes

5 eggs

8 ounces (225 g) reduced-fat cream cheese, softened

¼ cup (60 g) nonfat plain Greek yogurt

1 teaspoon salt

⅛ teaspoon ground black pepper

1 teaspoon Southwest-style seasoning

⅛ teaspoon red pepper flakes

¾ cup (120 g) chopped onions

1 pound (455 g) turkey sausage, cooked and crumbled

½ cup (60 g) Colby jack shredded cheese

» Spray your crock with nonstick cooking spray.

» Dump the potatoes into the crock.

» In a bowl, mix together the eggs, cream cheese, yogurt, salt, pepper, Southwest-style seasoning, and red pepper flakes. Stir in the onion, sausage, and cheese. Pour the egg mixture over the potatoes, and then stir it through.

» Cover the crock and cook on LOW for 7 to 8 hours or on HIGH for 3½ to 4 hours.

RECOMMENDED SLOW COOKER SIZE:
3 to 5 quart (3 to 5 L)

YIELD: 6 to 8 servings

Savory Egg-White Breakfast Bake

Light, yet delicious, this egg white breakfast bake filled with Gouda, spinach, and bacon tastes like a dish you would get at a trendy breakfast spot. It comes out light and fluffy and is incredibly easy to assemble.

2 cups (475 ml) egg whites

¾ cup (175 ml) almond milk

1 teaspoon fresh minced garlic

½ teaspoon sea salt

⅛ teaspoon ground black pepper

4 slices bacon, cooked and chopped

2 cups (60 g) spinach, torn

2 cups (225 g) shredded Gouda cheese

» Line your crock with parchment paper and spray it with nonstick cooking spray.

» In a bowl, mix together the egg whites, milk, garlic, salt, and pepper. Pour the mixture into the prepared crock.

» Sprinkle the egg mixture with the bacon, spinach, and then the cheese.

» Cover the crock and cook on LOW for 2 hours. (I do not recommend trying to cook this on HIGH.)

» Use the parchment paper to lift it out of the crock for easy cutting and serving.

RECOMMENDED SLOW COOKER SIZE:
5 to 7 quart (5 to 7 L)

YIELD: 6 to 8 servings

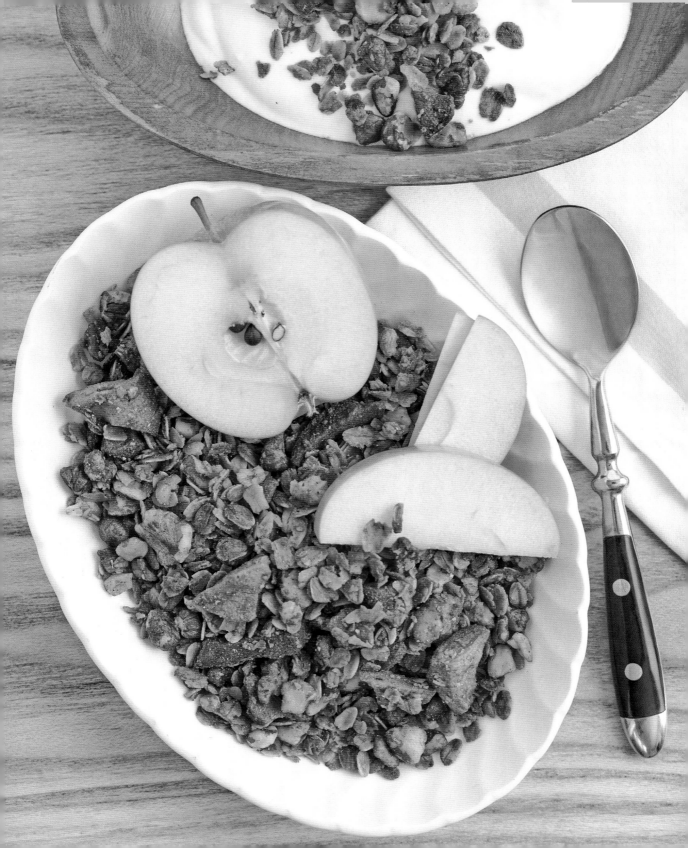

Apple Pie Granola

 DAIRY-FREE

If you love apple pie and you love granola, then this is for you. Adorned with pieces of dried apples, this granola will make you feel like you're eating an apple pie.

6 cups (480 g) old-fashioned oats

2 cups (60 ounces, or 1.7 kg) dehydrated apples

1 cup (120 g) chopped nuts of your choice, optional (pecans or walnuts are suggested)

½ cup (170 g) honey

½ cup (100 g) coconut oil, melted

2 teaspoons (5 g) apple pie spice

½ teaspoon cinnamon

» Spray your crock with nonstick cooking spray.

» Place all of the ingredients into the crock. Give it a good stir.

» Cover the crock and cook on LOW for 4 to 6 hours, stirring it frequently so it does not burn. (I do not recommend cooking this on HIGH.)

» Remove the granola from the crock and spread it out on parchment paper to cool. Store the granola in a tightly sealed container.

RECOMMENDED SLOW COOKER SIZE:
5 quart (5 L) or larger

YIELD: 16 to 20 servings

 TIPS & SUGGESTIONS

» This granola may be kept in the cupboard for 3 to 4 weeks in a tightly sealed container.
» To extend the life of your granola, you can keep it in the refrigerator.
» This would be wonderful on top of yogurt or ice cream or served like cereal with milk.

WAKE UP TO BREAKFAST

Cinnamon Maple Pecan Granola

The smell of cinnamon pecans alone is enough to make you drool. This granola has the wonderful flavor of cinnamon, pecans, and dried cherries, topped with the extra sweetness of maple syrup.

6 cups (480 g) old-fashioned oats

2 cups (220 g) chopped Cinnamon Sugar Pecans (see page 45)

1 cup (160 g) dried cherries

½ cup (65 g) sunflower seeds

¼ cup (45 g) flaxseed (optional)

½ cup (120 ml) maple syrup

½ stick butter (55 g), melted

½ teaspoon cinnamon

>> Spray your crock with nonstick cooking spray.

>> Add all of the listed ingredients. Give it a good stir.

>> Cover the crock and cook on LOW for 4 to 6 hours, stirring it frequently so it does not burn. (I do not recommend cooking this on HIGH.)

>> Remove the granola from the crock and spread it out on parchment paper to cool. Store the granola in a tightly sealed container.

RECOMMENDED SLOW COOKER SIZE:
5 quart (5 L) or larger

YIELD: 16 to 20 servings

TIPS & SUGGESTIONS

>> This granola should keep in the cupboard for 3 to 4 weeks in a tightly sealed container.

>> To add life to your granola, you can keep it in the refrigerator.

>> This would be wonderful on top of yogurt or ice cream or served like cereal with milk.

RECIPE NOTE

To make this recipe dairy-free, use coconut oil in place of the butter.

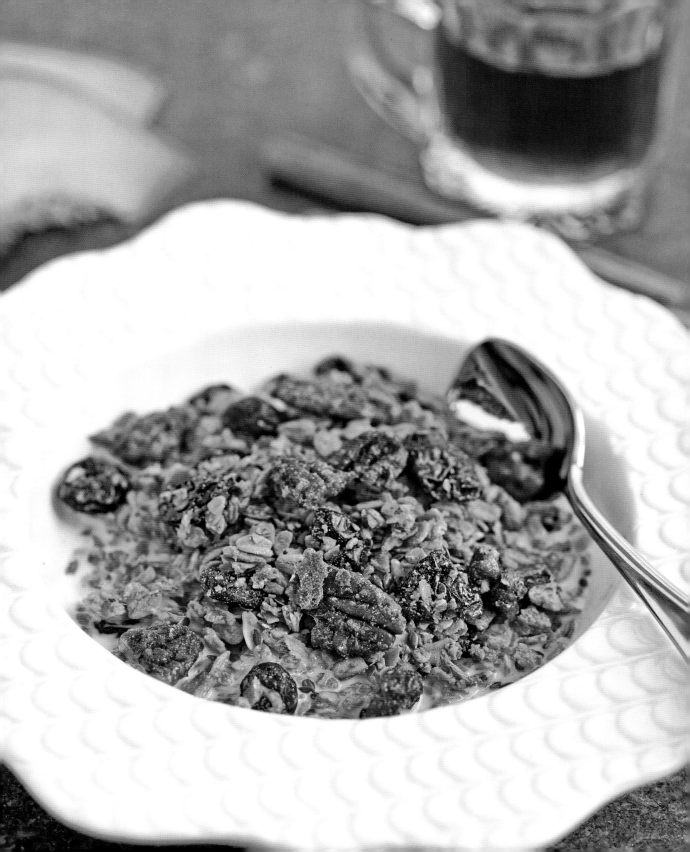

Vanilla Honey Walnut Granola

 DAIRY-FREE

There is nothing fancy about this granola, but it's still incredibly tasty. Made healthier with the use of the incredibly flavorful coconut oil, this no muss, no fuss granola will help you get your day off to an incredible start.

4 cups (320 g) old-fashioned oats
1½ cups (180 g) chopped walnuts
2 teaspoons (10 ml) vanilla
½ cup (170 g) honey
⅓ cup (60 g) coconut oil, melted
½ teaspoon cinnamon
⅛ teaspoon nutmeg

» Spray your crock with nonstick cooking spray.

» Add all of the listed ingredients. Give it a good stir.

» Cover the crock and cook on LOW for 4 to 6 hours, stirring it frequently so it does not burn. (I do not recommend cooking this on HIGH.)

» Remove the granola from the crock and spread it out on parchment paper to cool. Store the granola in a tightly sealed container.

RECOMMENDED SLOW COOKER SIZE:
3 to 5 quart (3 to 5 L)

YIELD: 10 to 16 servings

 ## TIPS & SUGGESTIONS

» **This granola should keep in the cupboard for 3 to 4 weeks in a tightly sealed container.**
» **To add life to your granola, you can keep it in the refrigerator.**
» **This would be wonderful on top of yogurt or ice cream or served like cereal with milk.**

Strawberry Rhubarb Steel Cut Oatmeal

 DAIRY-FREE

This is a creamy, sweet, tart oatmeal to help you start the day in a very healthy way. Sweet strawberries mixed with tart rhubarb give this a unique flavor, and it is a great alternative to the traditional plain ole' oatmeal.

1½ cups (120 g) steel cut oats
½ cup (100 g) turbinado sugar
¼ teaspoon apple pie spice
6 cups (1.4 L) coconut milk
1 teaspoon vanilla
1½ cups (385 g) frozen strawberries, chopped
2 rhubarb stalks or 1 cup (130 g) frozen rhubarb, chopped

» Spray your crock with nonstick cooking spray.

» Pour in the oats, sugar, and apple pie spice. Pour the milk and vanilla over the top and give a quick stir.

» Cover and cook on LOW for 8 hours or on HIGH for 4 hours. About 1 hour before it's done, stir in the strawberries and rhubarb.

RECOMMENDED SLOW COOKER SIZE:
3 quart (3 L)

YIELD: 6 servings

Banana Bread Oatmeal

 DAIRY-FREE

This oatmeal offers all of the yumminess of banana bread, but in oatmeal form. Seasoned with cinnamon, nutmeg, and with chunks of bananas, this oatmeal will stand apart from the rest.

1½ cups (120 g) steel cut oats
½ cup (115 g) brown sugar
½ teaspoon cinnamon
¼ teaspoon nutmeg
6 cups (1.4 L) almond milk
1 teaspoon vanilla
2 bananas, sliced
¼ cup (35 g) raisins

» Spray your crock with nonstick cooking spray.

» Pour in the oats, sugar, cinnamon, and nutmeg. Pour the milk and vanilla over the top and give a quick stir. Stir in the bananas and raisins last.

» Cover the crock and cook on LOW for 8 hours or on HIGH for 4 hours.

RECOMMENDED SLOW COOKER SIZE:
3 quart (3 L)

YIELD: 6 servings

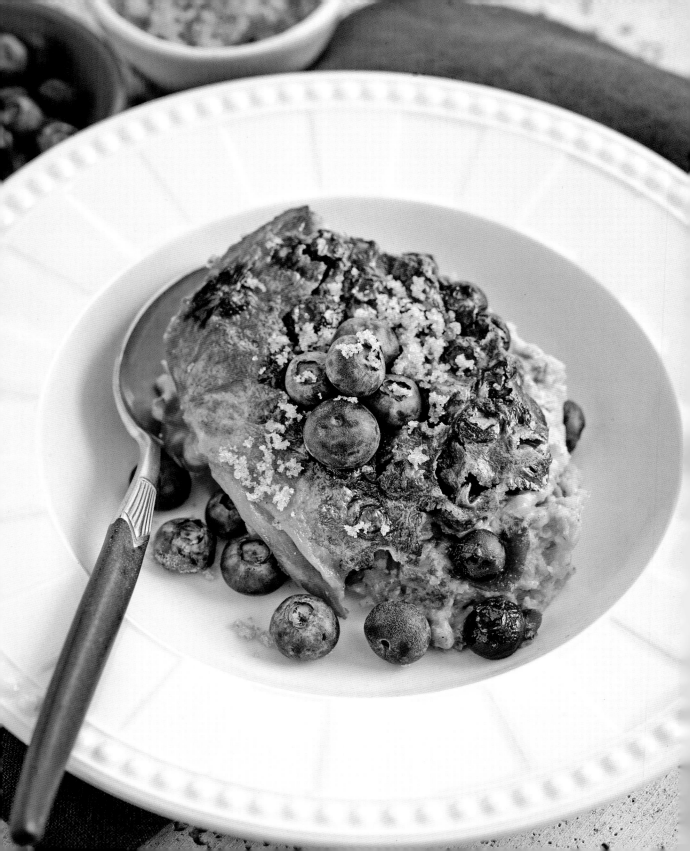

Blueberry Date Oatmeal

 DAIRY-FREE

Purple oatmeal? Yes please—especially when it comes from blueberries! The added sweetness of the dates makes this oatmeal a real crowd pleaser.

1½ cups (120 g) steel cut oats
½ cup (100 g) turbinado sugar
½ teaspoon cinnamon
6 cups (1.4 L) almond milk
1 teaspoon vanilla
1 cup (145 g) fresh blueberries
3 or 4 dates, pitted and diced

» Spray your crock with nonstick cooking spray. Pour in the oats, sugar, and cinnamon. Pour the milk and vanilla over the top and give a quick stir. Stir in the blueberries and dates last.

» Cover the crock and cook on LOW for 8 hours or on HIGH for 4 hours.

RECOMMENDED SLOW COOKER SIZE:
3 quart (3 L)

YIELD: 6 servings

 TIPS & SUGGESTIONS

» Serve this with fresh blueberries and a sprinkle of brown sugar on top as shown in the photo to make it extra special.
» You can change the flavor of this oatmeal by experimenting with different types of milk. Try coconut, cashew, vanilla-almond, or soy milk to change things up.

Cinnamon Roll Oatmeal

Finding gluten-free cinnamon rolls can be difficult. Making gluten-free cinnamon rolls takes way too much time. Making Cinnamon Roll Oatmeal is *simple* and *quick*! Drizzle your oatmeal with a delicious cinnamon frosting, and you've got a decadent dessert-like oatmeal for breakfast.

1½ cups (120 g) steel cut oats

½ cup (115 g) brown sugar

1½ teaspoons cinnamon

6 cups (1.4 L) almond milk

1 teaspoon vanilla

½ cup (115 g) cinnamon frosting, store-bought, or follow the frosting recipe on page 159, substituting cinnamon for the pumpkin pie spice.

» Spray your crock with nonstick cooking spray. Pour in the oats, sugar, and cinnamon. Pour the milk and vanilla over the top and give a quick stir.

» Cover the crock and cook on LOW for 8 hours or on HIGH for 4 hours.

» When you are ready to serve this, swirl in the cinnamon frosting.

RECOMMENDED SLOW COOKER SIZE:
3 quart (3 L)

YIELD: 6 servings

RECIPE NOTE

You can easily make this recipe dairy-free by replacing the cinnamon frosting with the following alternative: Mix together 1 cup (120 g) powdered sugar, 1 teaspoon vanilla, 2 tablespoons (30 ml) almond milk, and ½ teaspoon cinnamon.

TIPS & SUGGESTIONS

» If you don't like the thickness of your oatmeal in the morning, you can thin it out by adding a bit of milk when serving.

» You can change the flavor of this oatmeal by experimenting with different types of milk. Try coconut, cashew, vanilla-almond, or soy milk to change things up.

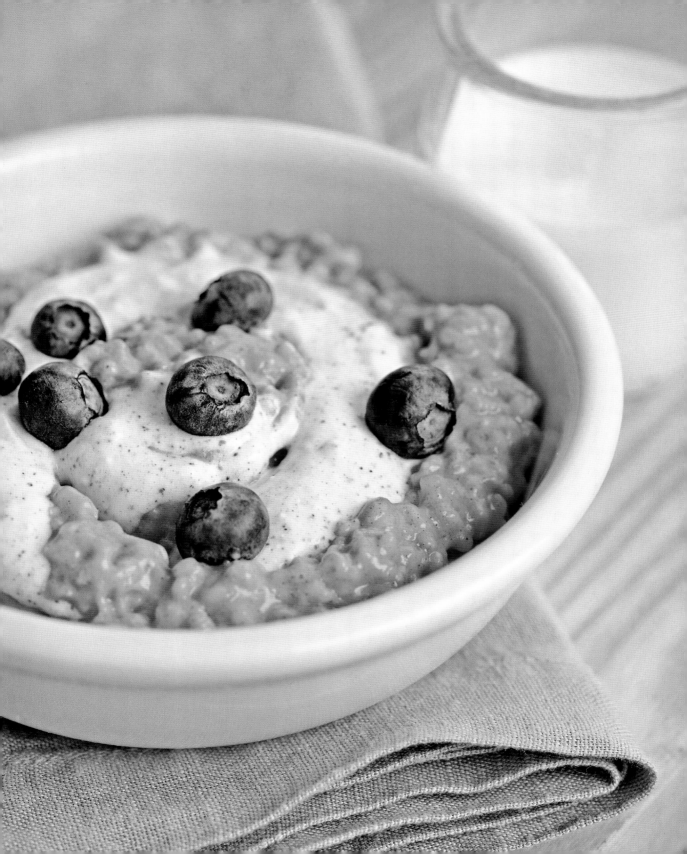

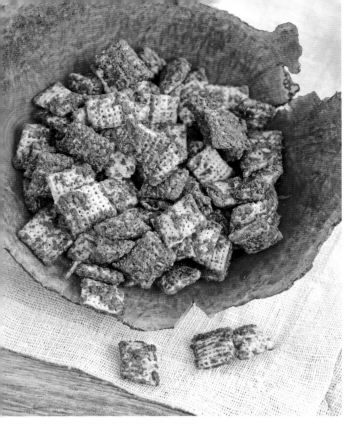

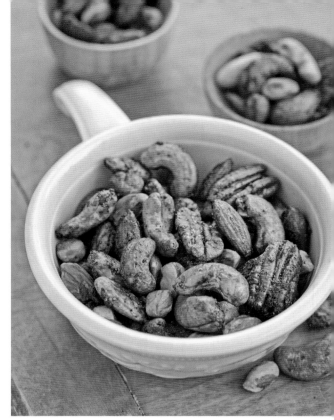

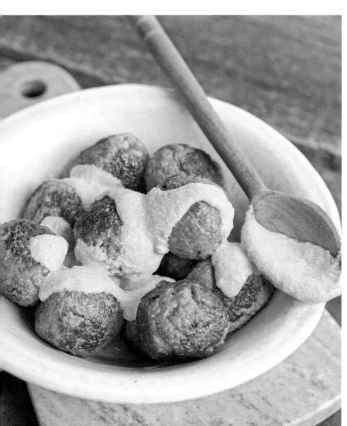

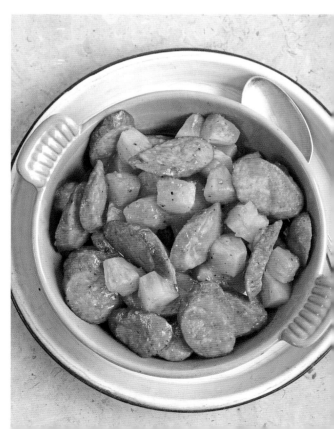

CHAPTER 3

STARTERS AND SNACKS THEY'LL WANT TO ATTACK!

Slow cookers can be used for other things besides dinner. Use your slow cooker to prepare delicious gluten-free snacks for your family, appetizing dips for you and your guests, and starters that people will be talking about for years to come.

DIPS

SNACKS

STARTERS

Buffalo Chicken Dip

If you love spicy buffalo chicken, then you'll love this dip. It has the perfect amount of that spiciness you crave, and with the chicken, it makes a very filling starter for any crowd.

8 ounces (225 g) boneless, skinless chicken breast

8 ounces (225 g) reduced-fat cream cheese, softened

1 cup (230 g) nonfat plain Greek yogurt

½ package (1 ounce, or 28 g) ranch seasoning

¾ cup (175 ml) wing sauce

1½ cups (175 g) shredded mozzarella cheese

½ cup (50 g) chopped red onion

» Spray your crock with nonstick cooking spray.

» Place the chicken in the bottom of the crock.

» In a bowl, mix together the cream cheese, Greek yogurt, ranch seasoning, wing sauce, mozzarella cheese, and onion. Pour the mixture over the top of the chicken.

» Cover the crock and cook on LOW for 5 to 6 hours or on HIGH for 2½ to 3 hours, stirring once or twice.

» Remove the chicken breast and shred it with two forks. Place the shredded chicken back into the sauce and stir it until it is well mixed.

RECOMMENDED SLOW COOKER SIZE:
2 quart (2 L)

YIELD: 15 to 20 servings

TIPS & SUGGESTIONS

This dip is amazing served with tortilla chips or with some gluten-free crostini.

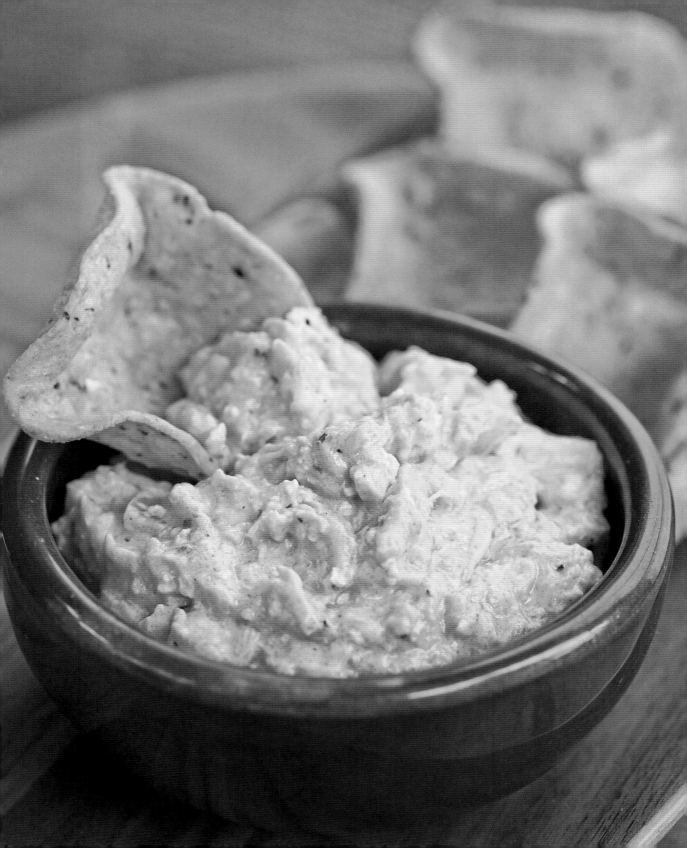

Cheesy Chorizo Dip

 INGREDIENTS OR LESS

Looking for something unexpected to serve to your guests? In my opinion, chorizo is one of the most overlooked meats. The sweetness and spiciness of the chorizo turns this cheesy dip into a tempting starter your guests will go crazy for.

1 package (12 ounces, or 340 g) Velveeta cheese
8 ounces (225 g) chorizo, cooked and crumbled
½ cup (130 g) salsa

» Spray your crock with nonstick cooking spray.

» Place all of the ingredients into your crock.

» Cover the crock and cook on LOW for 2 hours, or until it is completely melted. Once melted, stir and turn the slow cooker to WARM while serving. (I do not recommend cooking this on HIGH.)

RECOMMENDED SLOW COOKER SIZE:
2 quart (2 L)

YIELD: 8 to 12 servings

Chili con Queso Dip

 INGREDIENTS OR LESS

Forget the jar and grab a few simple ingredients to make your own chili con queso. The addition of fresh cilantro is what really makes this healthier version of chili con queso spectacular.

1 package (12 ounces, or 340 g) Velveeta cheese
8 ounces (225 g) ground beef, cooked and crumbled
½ can (15 ounces, or 425 g) kidney beans, rinsed and drained
¾ cup (195 g) salsa
¼ cup (4 g) chopped fresh cilantro

» Spray your crock with nonstick cooking spray.

» Place all of the ingredients into your crock.

» Cover the crock and cook on LOW for 2 hours, or until it is completely melted. Once melted, stir and turn the slow cooker to WARM while serving. (I do not recommend cooking this on HIGH.)

RECOMMENDED SLOW COOKER SIZE:
2 quart (2 L)

YIELD: 8 to 12 servings

TIPS & SUGGESTIONS

Either of these dips go great with gluten-free tortilla chips or pita.

Jalapeño Popper Dip

Miss not being able to indulge in breaded jalapeño poppers at restaurants? This dip will help cure that craving. Skip the breading and enjoy all of the deliciousness of jalapeño poppers, but as a dip for tortilla chips instead.

2 packages (8 ounces, or 225 g each) reduced-fat cream cheese, softened
1 cup (230 g) nonfat plain Greek yogurt
2 cans (4 ounces, or 115 g each) diced jalapeños
1½ cups (175 g) shredded Cheddar cheese
3 scallions, diced

» Spray your crock with nonstick cooking spray.

» Place all of the ingredients into your crock.

» Cover the crock and cook on LOW for 2 hours, or until it is completely melted. Once melted, stir and turn the slow cooker to WARM while serving. (I do not recommend cooking this on HIGH.)

RECOMMENDED SLOW COOKER SIZE:
2 quart (2 L)

YIELD: 15 to 20 servings

Pizza Dip

Pizza Dip is a real crowd pleaser. It has pretty much everything you put on your pizza, but in dip form.

2 packages (8 ounces, or 225 g, each) reduced-fat cream cheese
2 cans (15 ounces, or 425 g, each) pizza sauce
¼ pound (115 g) ground Italian sausage, cooked and crumbled
15 slices turkey pepperoni, chopped
½ cup (80 g) chopped onion
¼ cup (40 g) chopped green pepper
¼ cup (20 g) chopped mushrooms
1½ cups (175 g) shredded mozzarella cheese

» Spray your crock with nonstick cooking spray.

» Place the cream cheese in the crock. Pour the pizza sauce over the cream cheese. Add the sausage, pepperoni, onion, pepper, mushrooms, and cheese. Give it a stir.

» Cover the crock and cook on LOW for 4 hours or on HIGH for 2 hours.

RECOMMENDED SLOW COOKER SIZE:
2 quart (2 L)

YIELD: 15 to 20 servings

TIPS & SUGGESTIONS

Your "crew" will love this with some gluten-free bread crisps, bread sticks, or crackers.

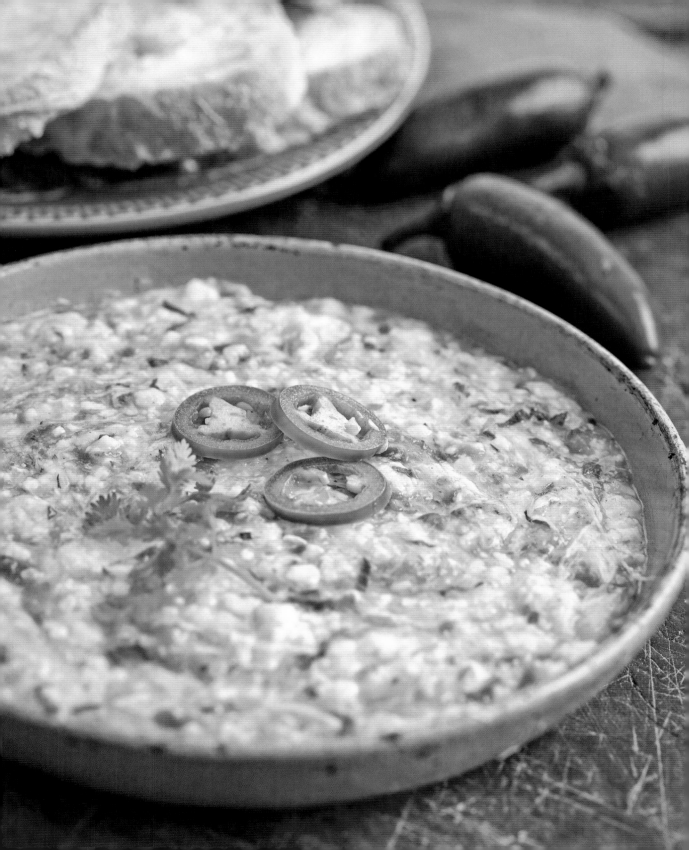

Queso Verde

 INGREDIENTS OR LESS

Verde means green, but don't let the color green scare you. With just five simple ingredients, it's creamy, cheesy, and delicious.

1 package (8 ounces, or 225 g) reduced-fat cream cheese

1 teaspoon fresh minced garlic

2 scallions, chopped finely

16 ounces (455 g) queso blanco cheese, shredded

1 jar (16 ounces, or 455 g) salsa verde

» Spray your crock with nonstick cooking spray.

» Place the cream cheese, garlic, and scallions in the crock. Place the queso blanco on top of that, and then pour the salsa verde over the top.

» Cover the crock and cook on LOW, stirring every hour for about 3 hours, or until everything is melted and combined. (The queso blanco doesn't get as smooth as most cheeses, so don't be worried if it's not 100 percent smooth. I do not recommend trying to cook these on HIGH.)

RECOMMENDED SLOW COOKER SIZE:
2 quart (2 L)

YIELD: 20 to 25 servings

 RECIPE NOTE

If you can't find queso blanco, don't panic. Just find another type of Mexican cheese at your grocery store. Most of the time, you will find these cheeses separate from the cheese case. I usually find the Mexican cheeses near the refrigerated tortillas. If you can't find them there, ask an associate at your local grocery store.

 TIPS & SUGGESTIONS

» This dip is wonderful with tortilla chips.

» It's also delicious on the Barbacoa Beef Burrito Bowls on page 95.

Spinach and Artichoke Dip

Talk about addicting! When you mix spinach and artichokes with cream cheese, Parmesan cheese, and fresh garlic, you make an incredibly delicious dip that you won't be able to stop eating.

1 cup (230 g) sour cream

1 can (15 ounces, or 425 g) artichoke hearts, drained and chopped

8 ounces (225 g) frozen spinach, thawed, liquid squeezed out

½ cup (50 g) grated Parmesan cheese

2 tablespoons (20 g) fresh minced garlic

1 teaspoon salt

¼ teaspoon ground black pepper

2 packages (8 ounces, or 225 g, each) nonfat or reduced-fat cream cheese, cubed

» Spray your crock with nonstick cooking spray.

» In the crock, mix together the sour cream, artichokes, spinach, Parmesan cheese, garlic, salt, and pepper. Stir the cream cheese into this mixture.

» Cover the crock and cook on LOW for 2 hours, or until it is completely melted. Once melted, stir and turn the slow cooker to WARM while serving. (I do not recommend cooking this on HIGH.)

RECOMMENDED SLOW COOKER SIZE: 2 quart (2 L)

YIELD: 12 to 16 servings

TIPS & SUGGESTIONS

» This dip is amazing with some gluten-free bread crisps, crostini, or tortilla chips.

» You can cool the leftovers and eat it as a cold spinach and artichoke dip the next day.

Cinnamon Sugar Pecans

 DAIRY-FREE

Your house will smell absolutely *amazing* while you're making these. These sweet cinnamon pecans will make a great snack or be an amazing addition to a recipe, such as the Cinnamon Maple Pecan Granola on page 28.

16 ounces (455 g) pecans
½ cup (115 g) brown sugar
½ cup turbinado sugar
1 tablespoon (7 g) cinnamon
1 teaspoon sea salt
1 tablespoon (12 g) coconut oil
1 egg white
2 teaspoons (10 ml) vanilla
2 tablespoons (28 ml) water

» Spray your crock with nonstick cooking spray.

» Place all of the ingredients into the crock and mix very well so everything is fairly evenly coated.

» Cover the crock and cook on LOW for 5 to 6 hours or on HIGH for 2½ to 3 hours. Stir the pecans every 40 to 60 minutes so they do not burn.

RECOMMENDED SLOW COOKER SIZE:
2 quart (2 L)

YIELD: 4 cups

 ## TIPS & SUGGESTIONS

» Let the pecans cool completely before storing them in an airtight container.
» The pecans should keep for a good month in a cool, dark place.

Hazelnut and Kahlua Rice Snack Mix

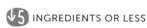 INGREDIENTS OR LESS

I had your attention at hazelnut and Kahlua, right? This sweet treat is the adult version of your old favorite childhood snack.

1 cup (260 g) chocolate-hazelnut spread, such as Nutella
½ cup (120 ml) Kahlua
1 teaspoon vanilla
¼ cup (45 g) milk chocolate chips
8 cups (215 g) gluten-free rice square cereal

» Spray your crock with nonstick cooking spray.

» Place the chocolate-hazelnut spread, Kahlua, vanilla, and chocolate chips into the crock.

» Cover the crock and cook on LOW for approximately 1½ hours or on HIGH for about 40 to 45 minutes, or until everything is melted together. Stir it. Pour in the rice square cereal and stir it all around.

» Lay parchment paper down on your counter and pour the rice cereal mixture onto it, spreading it out. Leave it there until it is dry.

» Store in an air-tight container. It should be good for about a week or two. It may lose its crunch after that.

RECOMMENDED SLOW COOKER SIZE:
5 to 7 quart (5 to 7 L)

YIELD: 10 to 15 servings

 TIPS & SUGGESTIONS

» Add to the sweetness of this recipe by adding your favorite candy to the mix after it cools.
» Sprinkle this with powdered sugar when finished for an extra-decadent treat.
» Try this recipe with RumChata or Bailey's Irish Cream instead of the Kahlua.

Sweet and Spicy Mixed Nuts

 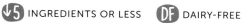 INGREDIENTS OR LESS   DAIRY-FREE

Nuts make a great snack, but these nuts stand out among the rest. They're a little bit sweet and a little bit spicy. These would be great to snack on all day, or to serve at a party.

4 cups (580 g) raw mixed nuts, such as almonds, pecans, cashews, and pistachios

1 teaspoon kosher salt

1 teaspoon curry powder

2 teaspoons (10 g) fiesta lime seasoning, such as Mrs. Dash brand

1 tablespoon (14 ml) maple syrup

» Spray your crock with nonstick cooking spray.

» Place nuts, spices, and maple syrup in the crock. Stir them up well so everything is coated evenly.

» Cover the crock and cook on LOW for 4 to 5 hours, or until slightly brown. Stir the nuts every 40 to 60 minutes to make sure they're not burning. (I do not recommend cooking this on HIGH.)

RECOMMENDED SLOW COOKER SIZE: 2 quart (2 L)

YIELD: 4 cups (580 g)

TIPS & SUGGESTIONS

» Let your nuts cool completely before storing them in a tightly sealed container.

» These should last for at least a good month in a cool, dark area.

» These would be a great addition to the Rice Square Snack Mix on page 49.

» Use whatever types of raw nuts you enjoy.

Asian Zing Wings

 DAIRY-FREE

These wings are sweet and spicy, and they have a hint of orange that will make your taste buds dance. Serve them at a party, or have wings for dinner one night. Either way, these will be some of the best wings you've ever had.

2 pounds (900 g) chicken wings, tips removed

¼ cup (85 g) honey

2 teaspoons (10 ml) soy sauce

2 teaspoons (10 ml) teriyaki sauce

1 teaspoon rice vinegar

1 teaspoon orange juice

1 teaspoon sriracha

½ teaspoon orange zest

¼ teaspoon ginger

» Spray your crock with nonstick cooking spray.

» Place the wings into the crock.

» In a bowl, combine the ingredients, (honey through ginger) for the sauce and pour it over the wings.

» Cover the crock and cook on LOW for 4 to 6 hours or on HIGH for 2 to 4 hours.

RECOMMENDED SLOW COOKER SIZE: 2 quart (2 L)

YIELD: 8 to 10 servings

RECIPE NOTE

If you like your sauce thicker, you can cook it on the stovetop. Cook the wings in the crock, seasoned with salt and pepper, remove them, and then toss them with the sauce you cooked on the stovetop just before serving.

Barbecue Teenie Weenies

 INGREDIENTS OR LESS   DAIRY-FREE

These little sausages make a quick and easy starter everyone will gobble up. With only four ingredients, it's an easy one to throw together.

1 bottle (12 ounces, or 340 g) sweet barbecue sauce

6 ounces (170 g) chili sauce

¼ cup (85 g) honey

2 packages (16 ounces, or 455 g, each) cocktail sausages

» Spray your crock with nonstick cooking spray.

» In the crock, mix together the barbecue sauce, chili sauce, and honey. Stir in the sausages.

» Cover the crock and cook on LOW for 2 hours, or until heated through, then turn to WARM while serving. (I do not recommend cooking this on HIGH.)

RECOMMENDED SLOW COOKER SIZE:
2 to 3 quart (2 to 3 L)

YIELD: 16 to 25 servings

Honey Barbecue Meatballs

 DAIRY-FREE

Everyone loves cocktail meatballs! These little guys won't disappoint, with their perfect combination of sweet and tangy.

FOR THE MEATBALLS:

1 pound (455 g) ground sirloin

1 egg

1 teaspoon dried minced onion

½ teaspoon salt

½ teaspoon garlic powder

⅛ teaspoon ground black pepper

¼ cup (30 g) gluten-free panko bread crumbs

FOR THE SAUCE:

1 can (8 ounces, or 225 g) tomato sauce

2 tablespoons (40 g) honey

2 tablespoons (28 ml) apple cider vinegar

1 tablespoon (15 g) brown sugar

⅛ teaspoon ground black pepper

» Spray your crock with nonstick cooking spray.

» **To make the meatballs:** Preheat the oven to 375°F (190°C, or gas mark 5).

» In a bowl, mix together all of the meatball ingredients and form them into about ½ to 1-inch (1 to 2 cm) balls. Place the meatballs on a rimmed baking sheet. Bake the meatballs for 15 to 20 minutes.

» **To make the sauce:** Pour the tomato sauce, honey, vinegar, brown sugar, and pepper into the crock and stir. Place the meatballs into the sauce.

» Cover the crock and cook on LOW for 5 to 6 hours or on HIGH for 2½ to 3 hours.

RECOMMENDED SLOW COOKER SIZE:
2 quart (2 L)

YIELD: 30 to 32 meatballs

Buffalo Chicken Meatballs

These buffalo chicken meatballs are a healthier alternative to the buffalo meatballs you can buy from the grocery store. Don't worry though, you won't miss them one bit. These are moist and super tasty, and they have the perfect amount of spiciness.

FOR THE MEATBALLS:

1½ pounds (680 g) ground chicken

½ cup (120 ml) hot sauce

2 tablespoons (10 g) dried minced onion

2 tablespoons (18 g) garlic powder

¼ teaspoon ground black pepper

1 egg

1 cup (115 g) gluten-free panko bread crumbs

1½ tablespoons (20 g) coconut oil or olive oil

1 cup (235 ml) chicken stock

FOR THE SAUCE:

2 cups (460 g) nonfat plain Greek yogurt

2 tablespoons (16 g) cornstarch

¼ cup (60 ml) hot sauce

» Spray your crock with nonstick cooking spray.

» **To make the meatballs:** In a bowl, combine the chicken, hot sauce, onion, garlic powder, pepper, egg, and bread crumbs. Mix this well and roll the mixture into 1½- to 2-inch (3 to 5 cm) balls.

» In a skillet, heat the oil over medium heat. Sear the meatballs on all sides, just so they hold together when you cook them. (You don't want to actually cook them because that's your slow cooker's job.)

» Place the seared meatballs into the crock and cover them with the stock.

» Cover the crock and cook the meatballs on LOW for 5 to 6 hours or on HIGH for 2½ to 3 hours.

» With a slotted spoon, remove the meatballs so you can work on your sauce.

» **To make the sauce:** In the crock, add the yogurt, cornstarch, and hot sauce to the juices already in there. Whisk it until well combined and add the meatballs back in. Cover the crock and cook on LOW for about another 30 to 45 minutes, or until the sauce is heated. (I do not recommend cooking this on HIGH.)

RECOMMENDED SLOW COOKER SIZE:
5 quart (5 L) or larger

YIELD: 18 to 24 servings

TIPS & SUGGESTIONS

» I suggest wearing disposable kitchen gloves when making this recipe. You don't want to get hot sauce all over your hands and then accidentally touch your eye or something!

» Serve the meatballs as an appetizer, or make them into a meal by serving them over rice or quinoa.

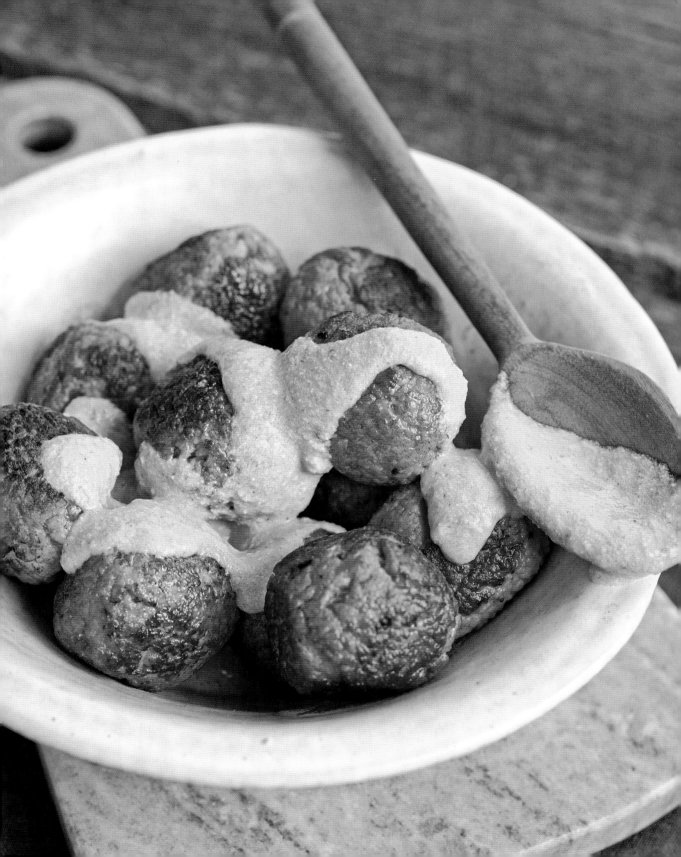

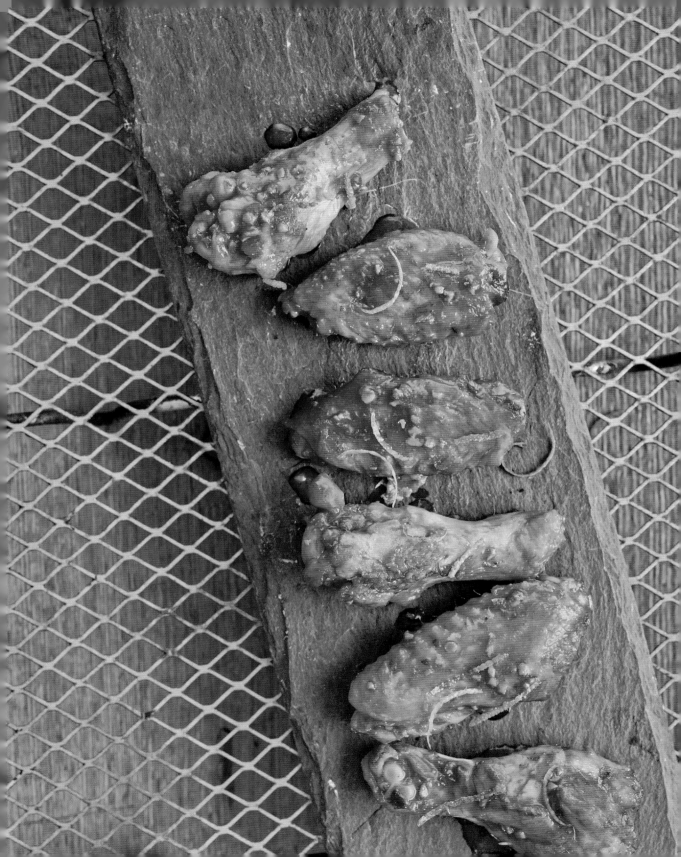

Chili Lime Wings

 DAIRY-FREE

Those wing places have nothing on these wings. The sweet, spicy, tangy sauce with the refreshing hint of lime makes these wings finger lickin' good!

2 pounds (900 g) chicken wings, tips removed

2 tablespoons (28 ml) chili sauce

1½ tablespoons (20 ml) lime juice

2 teaspoons (10 ml) teriyaki sauce

½ teaspoon soy sauce

½ teaspoon fresh minced garlic

3 tablespoons (40 g) turbinado sugar

½ teaspoon dried ginger

½ teaspoon lime zest

» Spray your crock with nonstick cooking spray.

» Place the wings into the crock.

» In a bowl, combine the ingredients, (chili sauce through lime zest), for the sauce and pour it over the wings.

» Cover the crock and cook on LOW for 4 to 6 hours or on HIGH for 2 to 4 hours.

RECOMMENDED SLOW COOKER SIZE:
2 quart (2 L)

YIELD: 8 to 10 servings

 ## RECIPE NOTE

If you like your sauce thicker, you can cook it on the stovetop. Cook the wings in the crock, seasoned with salt and pepper, remove them, and then toss them with the sauce you cooked on the stovetop just before serving.

Hawaiian Kielbasa Bites

 DAIRY-FREE

Adorned with bits of pineapple, these little kielbasa bites are easy to make and easy to become addicted to. The pineapple flavor really shines through, making this little appetizer a sweet and delightful appetizer the crowd will love.

1½ pounds (680 g) kielbasa, cut into bite-size pieces

1 can (8 ounces, or 225 g) tomato sauce

2 tablespoons (28 ml) apple cider vinegar

1 teaspoon Worcestershire sauce

¼ cup (60 g) brown sugar

⅛ teaspoon ground black pepper

3 tablespoons (45 ml) canned pineapple juice

1 can (20 ounces, or 565 g) pineapple chunks, juice separated and kept from the chunks

» Spray your crock with nonstick cooking spray.

» Place the kielbasa into the crock.

» In a bowl, mix together the tomato sauce, vinegar, Worcestershire sauce, sugar, pepper, and pineapple juice. Pour the mixture over the kielbasa.

» Cover the crock and cook on LOW for 3 to 4 hours. Add the pineapple chunks about 20 minutes before serving. (I do not recommend cooking this on HIGH.)

RECOMMENDED SLOW COOKER SIZE:
2 quart (2 L)

YIELD: 6 to 10 servings

 TIPS & SUGGESTIONS

You can make this into a whole meal by serving this over cooked white or brown rice, or quinoa.

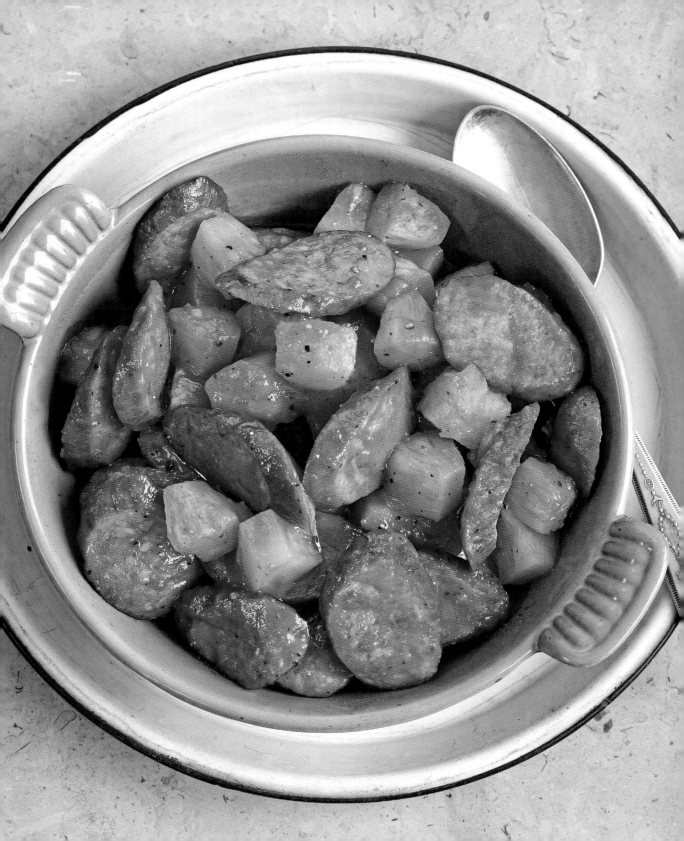

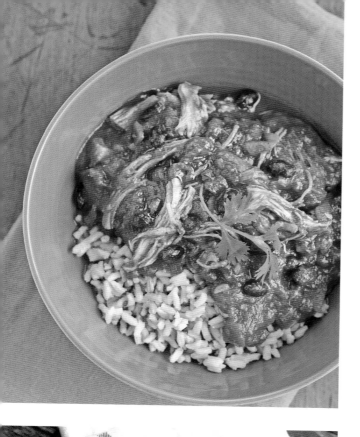
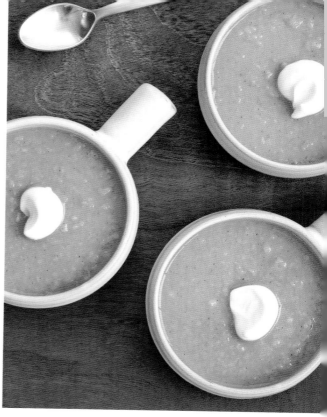
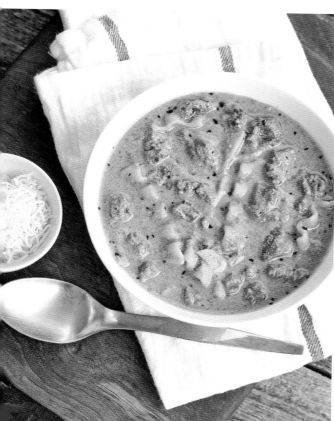
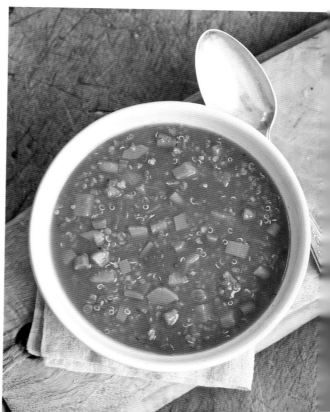

CHAPTER 4

SENSATIONAL SOUPS AND CHILIS

You don't have to wait for fall and winter to have soup. You can use your slow cooker year round to make some incredibly tasty soups for your family. Whether you're a meat-lover or a veggie-lover, or you just want to have alternatives to your "usual," this chapter has something for you.

Tomato Basil Chicken Stew

 DAIRY-FREE

This fragrant stew will please even the pickiest of eaters. Even though it's labeled as a stew, it has the versatility to be served a few different ways. Perk up those taste buds and try some of this fabulous tomato basil chicken stew.

3 pounds (1.4 kg) boneless, skinless chicken thighs, chopped into bite-size pieces

2 cups (220 g) cubed potatoes

1 can (28 ounces, or 795 g) crushed tomatoes

2 cans (14.5 ounces, or 410 g, each) diced tomatoes

1 can (6 ounces, or 170 g) tomato paste

½ cup (80 g) chopped onion

¼ cup (25 g) chopped celery

4 ounces (115 g) basil paste or 4 cups (160 g) fresh chopped basil

3 tablespoons (30 g) fresh minced garlic

4 cups (950 ml) chicken stock

» Spray your crock with nonstick cooking spray.

» Put the chicken and potatoes into the crock and pour the crushed tomatoes, diced tomatoes, tomato paste, onion, celery, basil paste or basil, and garlic over the top. Cover it with the stock and give it a stir.

» Cover the crock and cook on LOW for 8 to 9 hours or on HIGH for 4 to 4½ hours.

RECOMMENDED SLOW COOKER SIZE:
5 to 6 quart (5 to 6 L)

YIELD: 8 to 10 servings

 ## TIPS & SUGGESTIONS

» **This could be served over rice or gluten-free pasta.**
» **Add some cream at the end of cooking for an excellent creamy Tomato Basil Chicken Stew.**

Chicken and Lime Soup with Avocado Garnish

DF DAIRY-FREE

This is a light, brothy soup adorned with pieces of shredded chicken and flavored with a touch of lime. Top it with some fresh avocado, and you have an incredibly flavorful, yet light meal.

2 pounds (900 g) boneless, skinless chicken breasts

6 cups (1.4 L) unsalted chicken stock

1 can (14.5 ounces, or 410 g) diced tomatoes

1 cup (160 g) chopped red onion

½ cup (120 ml) lime juice

2 teaspoons (5 g) chili powder

2 teaspoons (12 g) sea salt

⅛ teaspoon ground black pepper

2 avocados, peeled, pitted, and diced

» Spray your crock with nonstick cooking spray.

» Place all of ingredients except for the avocado into the crock and give it a light stir.

» Cover the crock and cook on LOW for 6 to 7 hours or on HIGH for 3 to 3½ hours. Serve with the avocados on top.

RECOMMENDED SLOW COOKER SIZE:
5 to 6 quart (5 to 6 L)

YIELD: 4 to 6 servings

 TIPS & SUGGESTIONS

» If you're looking for a way to make this soup a bit heartier, serve it over ½ cup (80 g) cooked brown or white rice.

» You can easily make this recipe vegetarian by replacing the chicken with chickpeas and the chicken broth with vegetable broth.

Chicken Enchilada Soup

DF DAIRY-FREE

If you like enchiladas, you will love this soup. It has very simple ingredients and a great "kick" to it. Unlike typical enchiladas, no tortillas are involved. Instead, this delicious soup is served over a helping of rice.

1 can (15.5 ounces, or 445 g) black beans, rinsed and drained

1 can (14.5 ounces, or 410 g) diced tomatoes

1 can (10 ounces, or 280 g) enchilada sauce (mild or hot)

1 can (8 ounces, or 225 g) tomato sauce

1 can (6 ounces, or 170 g) tomato paste

2½ pounds (1.1 kg) boneless, skinless chicken breast, cut into bite-size pieces

1 cup (160 g) chopped onion

1 cup (235 ml) chicken stock

1 Anaheim pepper, diced

¼ teaspoon salt

¼ teaspoon ground black pepper

Cooked brown rice, for serving

» Spray your crock with nonstick cooking spray.

» Place the chicken in the crock with all of the remaining ingredients, except the rice.

» Cover the crock and cook on LOW for 6 to 7 hours or on HIGH for 3 to 3½ hours.

» When serving, place a helping of brown rice in the bottom of each bowl and ladle the soup over the top.

RECOMMENDED SLOW COOKER SIZE:
4 to 5 quart (4 to 5 L)

YIELD: 6 to 8 servings

TIPS & SUGGESTIONS

» Chop up a bit of fresh cilantro and serve it on top of each bowl of soup for special addition.

» If this soup isn't spicy enough for you, add some jalapeño slices on top.

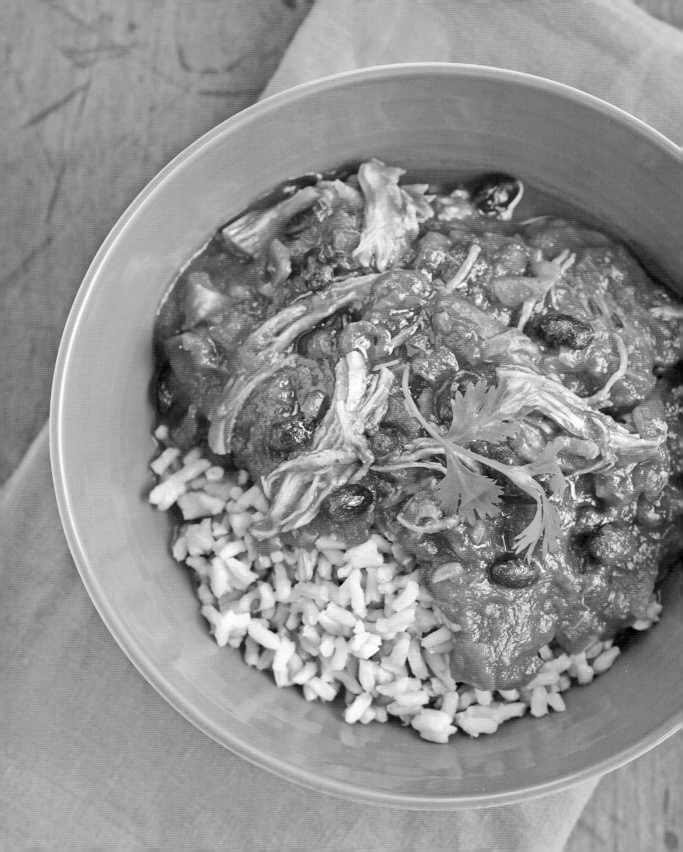

Tasty Turkey Chili with Sun-Dried Tomatoes

DF DAIRY-FREE

One of the things I love about chili is how it has so many variations. This tasty turkey chili includes the delicious and unexpected addition of sun-dried tomatoes. I think you'll find that everyone in your family will eat this crowd pleasing chili.

1 pound (455 g) ground turkey, cooked and crumbled

1 cup (160 g) chopped onion

2 teaspoons (6 g) fresh, minced garlic

½ cup (25 g) chopped sun-dried tomatoes

3 medium carrots, sliced into rounds

1 can (15.5 ounces, or 440 g) dark red kidney beans, rinsed and drained

1 bay leaf

1 tablespoon (7 g) onion powder

1 tablespoon (13 g) granulated sugar

2 teaspoons (5 g) chili powder

1 teaspoon ground mustard powder

½ teaspoon salt

½ teaspoon dried basil

½ teaspoon dried oregano

⅛ teaspoon ground black pepper

1 can (28 ounces, or 795 g) petite diced tomatoes

1 can (6 ounces, or 170 g) tomato paste

1 can (8 ounces, or 225 g) tomato sauce

2 cups (475 ml) chicken stock

» Spray your slow cooker with nonstick cooking spray.

» Place the turkey into the slow cooker and add the onion, garlic, sun-dried tomatoes, carrots, and kidney beans. Add the bay leaf, onion powder, sugar, chili powder, mustard powder, salt, basil, oregano, and pepper.

» Pour in the diced tomatoes with juice, tomato paste, tomato sauce, and stock.

» Cover the crock and cook on LOW for 7 to 8 hours or on HIGH for 3½ to 4 hours.

RECOMMENDED SLOW COOKER SIZE:
5 to 6 quart (5 to 6 L)

YIELD: 6 servings

TIPS & SUGGESTIONS

When serving this, sprinkle a little bit of shredded cheese on top with a dollop of sour cream. Some fresh chives on top would be lovely as well.

RECIPE NOTE

You can find sun-dried tomatoes in the produce section of your grocery store. I've found they are usually on one of the end-cap shelves. If you can't find it on your own, ask a sales associate at your store.

Irish Beef Stew

 DAIRY-FREE

This stew is super comforting, and it will warm you to the bone. With lots of good-for-you ingredients, you'll be fueling your body with the nutrients you need on a cold day—or any day, for that matter.

1½ pounds (680 g) leg of lamb, chopped into bite-size pieces

2 potatoes, peeled and diced

1 leek, chopped

2 cups (180 g) chopped cabbage

1 cup (130 g) chopped carrots

2 quarts (2 L) beef stock

2 cups (475 ml) water

2 sprigs fresh thyme

2 tablespoons (20 g) fresh minced garlic

2 teaspoons (12 g) salt

¼ teaspoon ground black pepper

½ cup (65 g) cornstarch

» Spray your crock with nonstick cooking spray.

» Place the lamb into the crock along with the potatoes, leek, cabbage, and carrots. Add the stock, water, thyme, garlic, salt, and pepper.

» Cover the crock and cook on LOW for 8 to 9 hours or on HIGH for 4 to 4½ hours.

» When the cook time is up, turn the slow cooker to HIGH, add the cornstarch, and stir well. Continue to let it cook until the stew reaches the desired thickness.

RECOMMENDED SLOW COOKER SIZE:
6 quart (6 L) or larger

YIELD: 10 to 12 servings

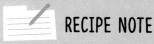

RECIPE NOTE

If you can't find lamb, beef will do just fine!

TIPS & SUGGESTIONS

You can make this stew even heartier by serving it over cooked brown or white rice, or quinoa.

Create-Your-Own Taco Soup

DF DAIRY-FREE

Make dinner interactive and fun with this super simple soup. Let the family make it their own by choosing toppings to add to their bowls. This type of meal is fun, and it satisfies even the pickiest eaters and the most adventurous eaters, too.

FOR THE TACO SEASONING:

4 tablespoons (30 g) chili powder

3 tablespoons (20 g) cumin

1 tablespoon (9 g) plus 2 teaspoons (6 g) garlic powder

1 tablespoon (7 g) plus 2 teaspoons (5 g) onion powder

2 teaspoons (12 g) salt

1 teaspoon dried oregano

1 teaspoon red pepper flakes

FOR THE SOUP:

1 jar (16 ounces, or 455 g) salsa (your favorite brand)

1 can (15.5 ounces, or 440 g) black beans, rinsed and drained

2½ tablespoons (7 g) taco seasoning (above)

6 cups (1.4 L) water

1 pound (455 g) lean ground beef, uncooked

SUGGESTED TOPPINGS:

Shredded cheese

Diced onions

Diced jalapeños

Plain Greek yogurt or sour cream

Tortilla chips

» **To make the taco seasoning:** Mix all of the spices together and store in an airtight container; 2½ tablespoons (25 g) of this mix equals one store-bought package of taco seasoning.

» **To make the soup:** Spray your crock with nonstick cooking spray.

» In the crock, place the salsa, black beans, taco seasoning, and water. Crumble in the ground beef.

» Cover the crock and cook on LOW for 7 to 8 hours or on HIGH for 3½ to 4 hours. Let the family add their own flair to their soup by adding whatever toppings they like best.

RECOMMENDED SLOW COOKER SIZE:
5 to 6 quart (5 to 6 L)

YIELD: 6 to 8 servings

RECIPE NOTE

It's always a great idea to have a batch or two of homemade taco seasoning in the cupboard. You won't ever have to reach for a packet of store-bought taco seasoning again.

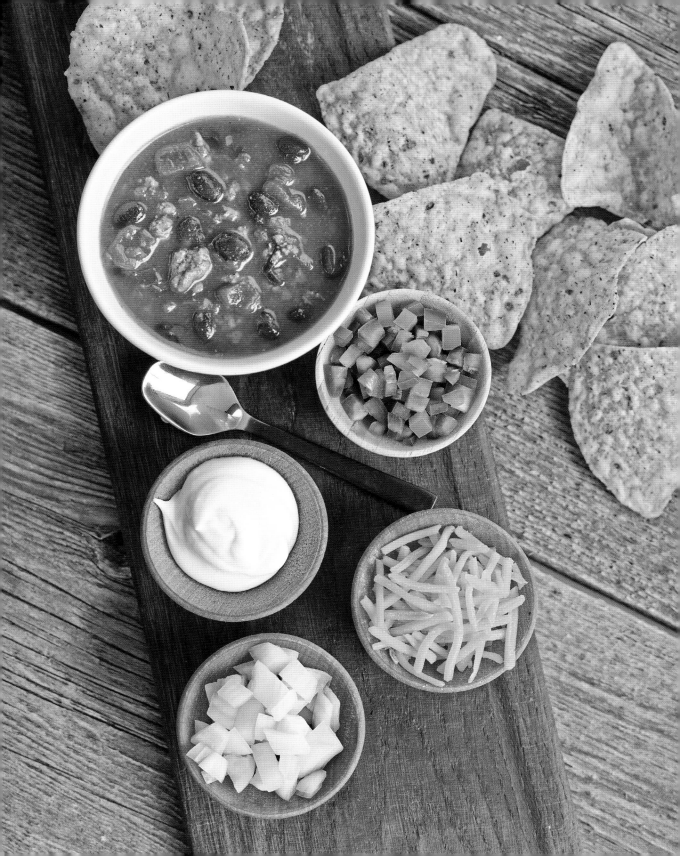

Beef Bourguignon

 DAIRY-FREE

Beef Bourguignon is pretty much a classic dish, so you definitely can't go wrong with this one. The pinot noir and cognac, together with the herbs and veggies, give this dish a depth of flavor that's incredible.

2½ to 3 pounds (1.1 to 1.4 kg) stew meat

2 medium onions, halved and sliced

1 bag (14.4 ounces, or 410 g) frozen pearl onions

6 ounces (170 g) variety of mushrooms (I like shitake, oyster, and baby bella.)

2 or 3 carrots roughly chopped

1 can (6 ounces, or 170 g) tomato paste

3 tablespoons (30 g) fresh minced garlic

1 tablespoon (2 g) minced fresh thyme

2 teaspoons (12 g) salt

1 bay leaf

32 ounces (945 ml) beef stock

1 bottle (750 ml) pinot noir

½ cup (120 ml) cognac

» Spray your crock with nonstick cooking spray.

» Place the stew meat into the crock, topped with the sliced onions, pearl onions, mushrooms, carrots, tomato paste, garlic, thyme, salt, and bay leaf.

» Pour the beef stock, pinot noir, and cognac into the crock and give it a good stir.

» Cover the crock and cook on LOW for 8 to 10 hours or on HIGH for 4 to 5 hours.

RECOMMENDED SLOW COOKER SIZE:
6 quart (6 L) or larger

YIELD: 8 to 10 servings

 RECIPE NOTE

If you're an alcohol-free family, you can replace the alcohol with beef broth. The flavor will be different, but delicious nonetheless.

Black Bean Soup

 DAIRY-FREE

This soup is light, simple, and flavorful. Packed with lots of black beans, tomatoes, onions, garlic, and some common spices, you'll have dinner ready to go in no time at all.

2 cans (15 ounces, or 425 g, each) black beans, rinsed and drained

1 can (14.5 ounces, or 410 g) diced tomatoes

½ cup (80 g) chopped onion

3 tablespoons (30 g) minced garlic

1 teaspoon sea salt

1 teaspoon tomato basil garlic seasoning, such as Mrs. Dash brand

½ teaspoon dried basil

¼ teaspoon ground black pepper

1 bay leaf

6 cups (1.4 L) vegetable stock

» Spray your crock with nonstick cooking spray.

» Place all of the ingredients into the crock.

» Cover the crock and cook on LOW for 6 to 7 hours or on HIGH for 3 to 3½ hours.

RECOMMENDED SLOW COOKER SIZE:
5 to 6 quart (5 to 6 L)

YIELD: 8 to 10 servings

RECIPE NOTE

For a more budget-friendly alternative, you can replace the canned black beans with dry beans. You will need to soak 1 cup (250 g) of dry black beans overnight in water. Drain and rinse before adding to the recipe.

Chickpea and Sweet Potato Curry Soup

DF DAIRY-FREE

Want to serve your family something very unexpected for dinner? This is it! This soup is filling and healthy, and it has delicious Indian flavors that will surprise and delight you.

2 medium sweet potatoes, peeled and diced

2 cans (15 ounces, or 425 g, each) garbanzo beans (chickpeas), rinsed and drained

¾ cup (120 g) chopped onion

2 tablespoons (25 g) coconut oil

1 tablespoon (10 g) fresh minced garlic

1 tablespoon (6 g) curry powder

1½ teaspoons garam masala

1 teaspoon turmeric

¼ teaspoon cayenne pepper

¼ cup (60 ml) lime juice

3 cups (700 ml) vegetable stock

» Spray your crock with nonstick cooking spray.

» Place the potatoes, beans, onion, oil, garlic, curry, garam masala, turmeric, and cayenne pepper into the crock. Cover them with the lime juice and stock.

» Cover the crock and cook on LOW for 7 to 8 hours or on HIGH for 3½ to 4 hours.

» When the soup is ready, use an immersion blender to purée it. If you do not have an immersion blender, carefully place a couple ladles of soup into a blender or cover the lid with a towel. Blend it until you reach your desired smoothness. (Be very careful! You don't want to be sprayed with hot liquid.)

RECOMMENDED SLOW COOKER SIZE:
3 to 4 quart (3 to 4 L)

YIELD: 6 to 10 servings

RECIPE NOTE

Garam masala is a spice blend that may be found in the spice aisle of your grocery store or at an Indian grocer.

TIPS & SUGGESTIONS

Serve each bowl with a dollop of sour cream or nonfat plain Greek yogurt for extra creaminess. It also adds a beautiful contrast in color.

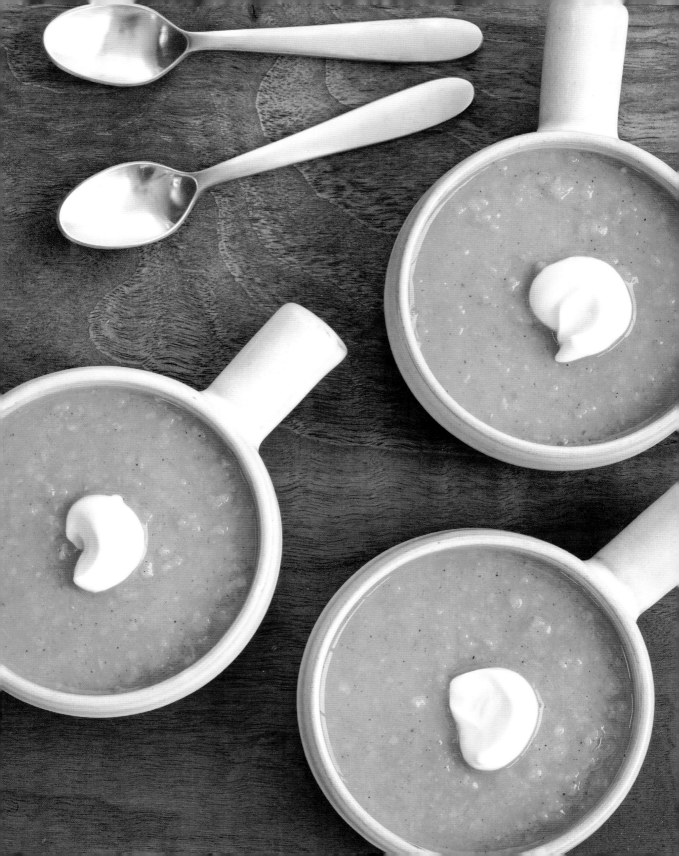

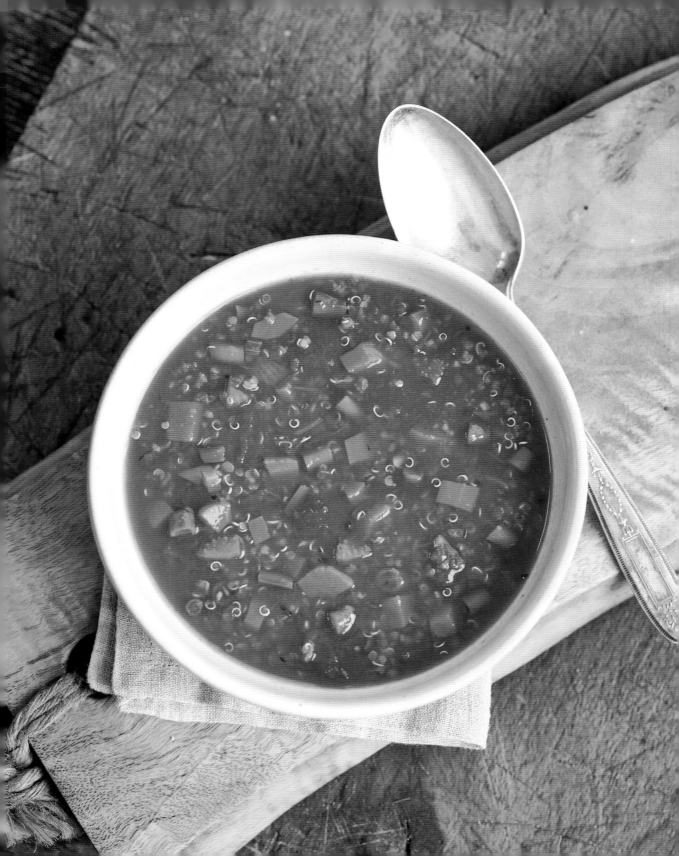

Quinoa Minestrone

 DAIRY-FREE

This soup is packed full of nutrition with carrots, celery, and fresh green beans. It has just a hint of spiciness, and the quinoa adds just the perfect texture to this delicious soup. You won't miss the noodles, I promise.

¾ cup (130 g) quinoa, rinsed

¼ cup (40 g) chopped onion

1 cup (100 g) fresh green beans, cut into
   ½-inch (1 cm) pieces

1 cup (130 g) chopped carrots

½ cup (50 g) chopped celery

1 can (14.5 ounces, or 410 g) diced tomatoes

1 can (14 ounces, or 395 g) crushed tomatoes

2 teaspoons (12 g) salt

1 teaspoon dried oregano

1 teaspoon dried basil

¼ teaspoon ground black pepper

6 cups (1.4 L) vegetable stock

» Spray your crock with nonstick cooking spray.

» Place the quinoa, onion, green beans, carrots, and celery into the crock. Pour the diced tomatoes and crushed tomatoes over the top. Add the salt, oregano, basil, and pepper, and then pour the stock over the top.

» Cover the crock and cook on LOW for 5 to 6 hours or on HIGH for 2½ to 3 hours.

RECOMMENDED SLOW COOKER SIZE:
4 to 5 quart (4 to 5 L)

YIELD: 6 to 8 servings

 ## TIPS & SUGGESTIONS

» You can add or delete any other vegetables you would like to this soup to make it your own.

» To make this a more traditional minestrone, instead of adding the quinoa in the beginning, cook some gluten-free pasta on the stovetop. When you're ready to serve, spoon some the pasta into each bowl and ladle the minestrone over the top.

Puréed Garlicky Chickpea and Vegetable Soup

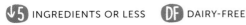 INGREDIENTS OR LESS DAIRY-FREE

Don't let this soup fool you! Five ingredients doesn't mean it's lacking flavor. This soup is incredibly flavorful, smooth, and sweet.

2½ cups (585 ml) vegetable stock

2 cups (480 g) canned garbanzo beans (chickpeas), rinsed and drained

1 cup (90 g) sliced leeks

1 cup (150 g) fresh shelled peas

5 cloves garlic, chopped

» Spray your crock with nonstick cooking spray.

» Place all of the ingredients into your crock.

» Cover the crock and cook on LOW for 5 to 6 hours. (I do not recommend cooking this on HIGH.)

» Before serving, using an immersion blender, purée the soup until smooth.

RECOMMENDED SLOW COOKER SIZE:
4 to 5 quart (4 to 5 L)

YIELD: 6 servings

 ## RECIPE NOTE

This recipe was made with minimal ingredients for your convenience. To add even more flavor to this soup, you could add additional vegetables such as celery, carrots, and onions.

Quinoa Chili

 DAIRY-FREE

This chili is absolutely delicious. It is so fulfilling, I promise you won't miss the meat. Don't be fooled by the long list of ingredients either. It's a matter of opening a bunch of cans, chopping a few vegetables, and adding some spices. Easy peasy.

1 can (15.5 ounces, or 440 g) black beans, rinsed and drained

1 can (15.5 ounces, or 440 g) Great Northern beans, rinsed and drained

1 can (28 ounces, or 795 g) diced tomatoes

1 can (12 ounces, or 340 g) tomato paste

¾ cup (120 g) chopped onion

¾ cup (100 g) chopped carrots

1 cup (70 g) chopped baby bella mushrooms

1 cup (175 g) quinoa, uncooked, rinsed

2 tablespoons (18 g) garlic powder

1 tablespoon (7 g) onion powder

2 teaspoons (5 g) chili powder

1 teaspoon salt

1 teaspoon dried basil

1 teaspoon fiesta lime seasoning, such as Mrs. Dash brand

¼ teaspoon cumin

⅛ teaspoon ground black pepper

1 bay leaf

7 to 8 cups (1.6 to 2 L) water

>> Spray your crock with nonstick cooking spray.

>> Place all of the ingredients into your slow cooker, adding the water last. Give it a few stirs to mix up the tomato paste a bit with the water.

>> Cover the crock and cook on LOW for 8 to 9 hours or on HIGH for 4 to 4½ hours.

RECOMMENDED SLOW COOKER SIZE: 6 quart (6 L) or larger

YIELD: 8 to 10 servings

Super Healthy Cabbage Soup

 DAIRY-FREE

Don't let the word *healthy* fool you into thinking this isn't delicious, because it definitely is. This cabbage soup is packed full of cabbage, celery, carrots, onions, and of course, my own version of V8 juice without the added sodium. You can have multiple bowls of this without feeling any guilt at all.

3 cups (270 g) chopped cabbage

1½ cups (240 g) chopped onion

2 large tomatoes, chopped

3 carrots, halved and sliced

1 jalapeño pepper, seeded and diced

1 tablespoon (9 g) garlic powder

2 to 3 teaspoons (12 to 18 g) salt

1 teaspoon dried basil

1 teaspoon dried oregano

¼ teaspoon ground black pepper

1 can (46 ounces, or 1.4 L) no-salt-added tomato juice

5 cups (1.2 L) water

» Spray your crock with nonstick cooking spray.

» Place the cabbage, onion, tomatoes, carrots, and jalapeño pepper into the crock; top with the garlic powder, salt, basil, oregano, and black pepper. Pour in the tomato juice and water last. No need to stir!

» Cover the crock and cook on LOW for 8 hours or on HIGH for 4 hours.

RECOMMENDED SLOW COOKER SIZE:
5 quart (5 L) or larger

YIELD: 6 to 10 servings

 ## TIPS & SUGGESTIONS

» Want to turn this cabbage soup into a stuffed-cabbage soup? Serve it over cooked white or brown rice and you'll have a brand new alternative!

» If you don't like to work with fresh jalapeños, add a can of diced, mild jalapeños instead.

Tomato Lentil Soup

This soup offers all of the wonderfulness of creamy tomato soup, but with the addition of delicious lentils. A little bit of cumin and chili powder give this soup just a hint of spiciness, but the addition of unsweetened almond milk and nonfat plain Greek yogurt cool it down perfectly.

2 cups (360 g) red lentils

1 can (15.5 ounces, or 440 g) Great Northern beans, rinsed and drained

1 can (28 ounces, or 795 g) crushed tomatoes

1 can (16 ounces, or 445 g) tomato sauce

2 cups (320 g) minced red onion

2 tablespoons (18 g) garlic powder

1½ teaspoons chili powder

1½ teaspoons salt

1½ teaspoons cumin

1½ teaspoons paprika

5 cups (1.2 L) vegetable stock

2 cups (475 ml) unsweetened almond milk

Nonfat plain Greek yogurt, for garnish

» Spray your crock with nonstick cooking spray.

» Place the lentils, beans, tomatoes, tomato sauce, onion, garlic powder, chili powder, salt, cumin, paprika, and stock into the crock and give it a stir.

» Cover the crock and cook on LOW for 8 hours or on HIGH for 4 hours.

» At this point, if you wish to make the soup smoother, use an immersion blender and purée it for a bit, or you can leave it the way it is. It's really up to you and your desired preference. Either way, ladle 2 cups (475 ml) of the soup into a bowl and slowly add in the milk, stirring constantly. (This is how you temper the almond milk so your soup doesn't curdle when you add it.)

» Pour the tempered milk into the crock and stir well. Let it cook for another 15 to 20 minutes, just so the temperature comes back up. Serve each bowl with a dollop of yogurt on top.

RECOMMENDED SLOW COOKER SIZE:
4 to 5 quart (4 to 5 L)

YIELD: 6 to 8 servings

White Bean Chili

This chili is so simple, yet it's so incredibly tasty. Navy beans, cheese, onions, salsa, and a few simple spices turn this chili into something everyone will want you to make time and time again.

2 cups (500 g) dried navy beans, uncooked

14 cups (3.3 L) water, divided

1 jar (16 ounces, or 455 g) salsa (whatever brand and heat level you like)

1 cup (160 g) chopped onion

1 tablespoon (7 g) cumin

½ teaspoon salt

½ teaspoon ground black pepper

4 cups (940 ml) vegetable stock

1 block (7 ounces, or 200 g) pepper jack cheese, grated

1 block (7 ounces, or 200 g) Monterey jack cheese, grated

» In a large bowl, 8 to 12 hours before you are ready to make this soup, soak the navy beans in 12 cups (2.8 L) of water. When the time is up, rinse and drain the beans thoroughly.

» Spray your crock with nonstick cooking spray.

» Place the beans, salsa, onion, cumin, salt, and pepper into the crock. Pour the stock and the remaining 2 cups (475 ml) of water in last.

» Cover the crock and cook on LOW for 8 to 10 hours or on HIGH for 4 to 5 hours. When the cook time is over, turn your slow cooker to HIGH and add in the pepper jack cheese and Monterey jack cheese. Cook for an additional hour, or until the cheese is completely melted.

RECOMMENDED SLOW COOKER SIZE:
5 quart (5 L) or larger

YIELD: 6 to 8 servings

TIPS & SUGGESTIONS

Feel like chicken instead of beans? Add about 2 pounds (900 g) of boneless, skinless chicken breast instead of the beans, swap out the vegetable stock for chicken stock, and cook for only 6 hours on LOW or 3 hours on HIGH. Remove the chicken from the soup, shred it, and place it back into the soup before adding the cheese.

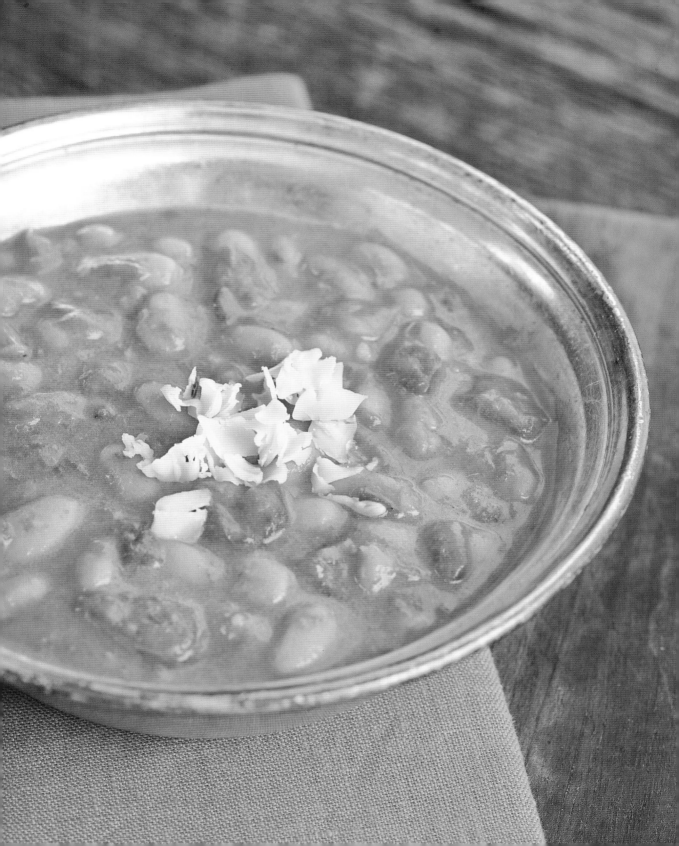

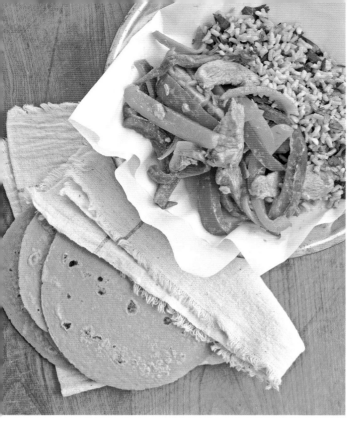
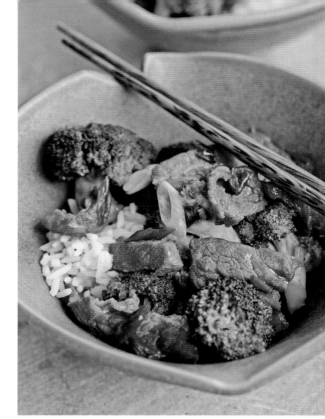
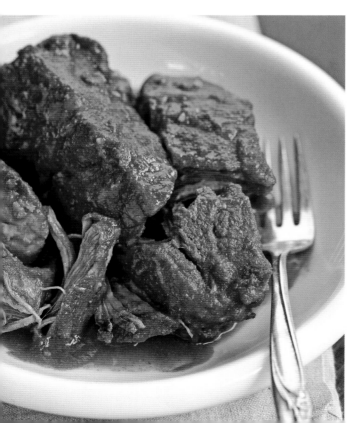
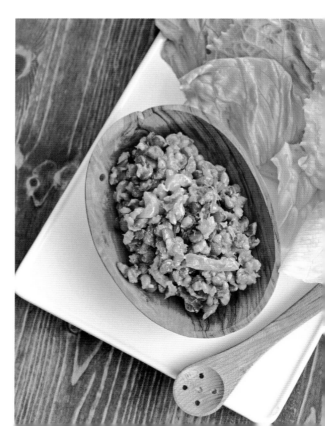

CHAPTER 5

MOUTHWATERING MAIN COURSES

You'll be surprised at what your slow cooker can make while you're away all day. Enjoy a vast selection of easy, gluten-free main course recipes anyone can make. You'll even find some recipes you can throw in last minute, with just a few simple ingredients.

Apple and Onion Pork Loin

 DAIRY-FREE

This smells amazing while it's cooking, and it tastes amazing, too. With a simple rub, some apples and onions, you'll turn a regular pork loin into something spectacular.

FOR THE RUB:

2 teaspoons (6 g) garlic powder

2 teaspoons (5 g) dried minced onion

1 teaspoon dried sage

1 teaspoon dried thyme

1 teaspoon dried rosemary

¾ teaspoon salt

FOR THE PORK:

3 pounds (1.4 kg) boneless pork loin

2 to 3 tablespoons (28 to 45 ml) olive oil

1½ to 2 cups (240 to 320 g) sliced sweet onion

3 to 4 cups (330 to 440 g) sliced apples

½ cup (120 ml) chicken stock

» **To make the rub:** In a small bowl, mix together all of the ingredients for the rub.

» **To make the pork:** Spray your crock with nonstick cooking spray. Place the pork in the crock and rub it on all sides with the oil. Press in the rub on all sides by sprinkling it on and pressing it onto the meat with your fingers.

» Place the onion and apples on top and around the pork, and then pour the stock around the pork.

» Cover the crock and cook on LOW for 7 to 8 hours or on HIGH for 3½ to 4 hours.

RECOMMENDED SLOW COOKER SIZE:
3 to 4 quart (3 to 4 L)

YIELD: 4 to 6 servings

 ## TIPS & SUGGESTIONS

Serve this with the Brown Sugar Mashed Sweet Potatoes on page 130 and the Sweet Acorn Squash on page 135.

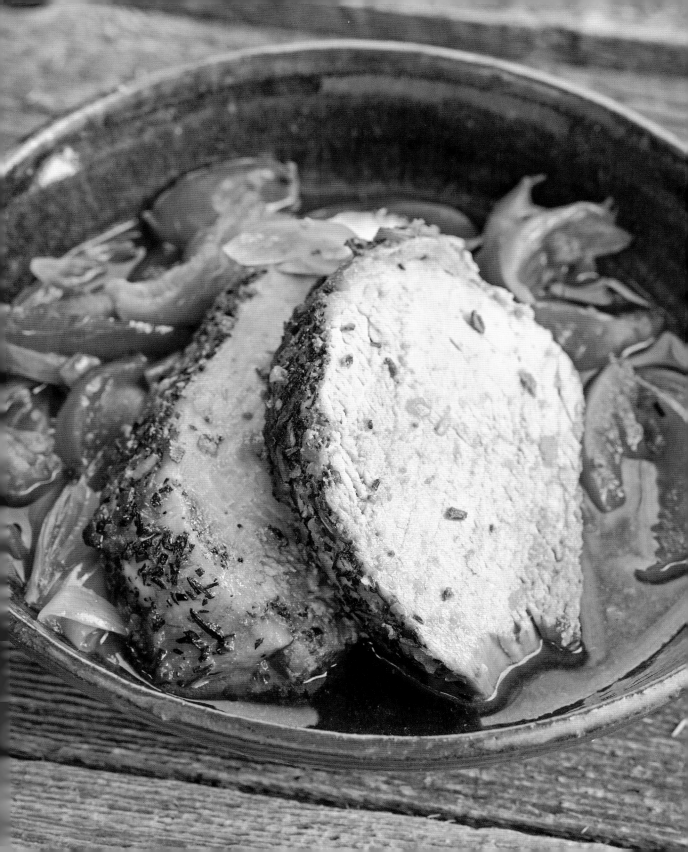

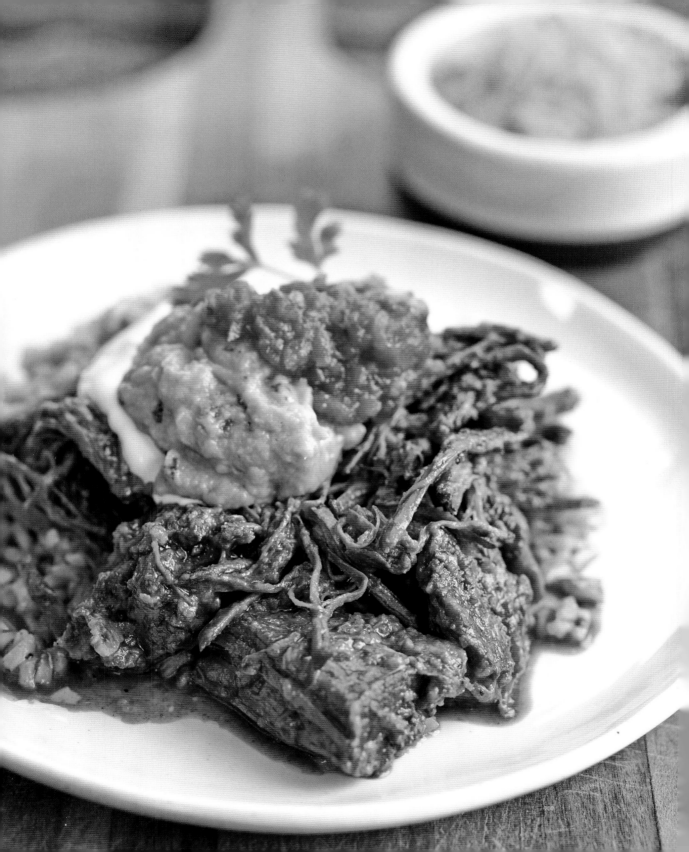

Barbacoa Beef Burrito Bowls

You'll think you've gone to a fiesta when you taste these Barbacoa Beef Burrito Bowls. This perfectly seasoned shredded beef served over flavorful lime rice with your favorite toppings make this a memorable meal you'll want to have time and time again. Enhance the flavor by serving the Queso Verde on page 43 over the top.

FOR THE BEEF:

2½ to 3 pounds (1.1 to 1.4 kg) chuck roast
½ cup (120 ml) chicken stock
½ cup (120 ml) apple cider vinegar
¼ cup (60 ml) lime juice
2 chipotle peppers in adobo sauce, diced, plus 1 teaspoon adobo sauce
2 bay leaves
3 tablespoons (20 g) cumin
2 teaspoons (12 g) salt
1 teaspoon dried oregano
¼ teaspoon ground black pepper

FOR THE RICE:

2 cups (330 g) cooked brown rice
1 tablespoon (14 g) butter, melted
¼ teaspoon salt
⅛ teaspoon ground black pepper
Lime juice, to taste

SUGGESTED TOPPINGS:

Shredded cheese
Sour cream or plain Greek yogurt
Guacamole
Salsa
Cilantro
Chopped onions

» To make the beef: Spray your crock with nonstick cooking spray.

» Place the chuck roast into the crock and add all of the remaining ingredients for the beef.

» Cover the crock and cook on LOW for 8 to 10 hours or on HIGH for 4 to 5 hours. Remove the beef from the crock, shred it, and then stir it back through the juices in the crock.

» To make the rice: In a bowl, mix together the rice, butter, salt, and pepper. Slowly add the lime juice, tasting along the way, until it has the right amount of "limeyness" to satisfy your taste buds.

» To serve, put some lime rice in a bowl and place some beef over the top. Add any suggested toppings you wish.

RECOMMENDED SLOW COOKER SIZE:
5 to 6 quart (5 to 6 L)

YIELD: 6 to 8 servings

RECIPE NOTE

You can find chipotles in adobo sauce in the international food aisle of your grocery store near the jalapeños and diced green chilies.

Chicken Caprese Bake

One of my favorite summertime snacks is tomato slices with fresh mozzarella, basil, with a drizzle of balsamic vinegar on top. So, I thought to myself, why not turn this in to a delicious meal? So I did! This chicken is incredibly flavorful and absolutely satisfying. This would be an impressive dish to serve to company to knock their socks off.

¾ cups (175 ml) balsamic vinegar

1 tablespoon (15 ml) olive oil

2 tablespoons (20 g) fresh minced garlic

1 teaspoon salt

¼ teaspoon ground black pepper

3 to 4 pounds (1.4 to 1.8 kg) boneless, skinless chicken breasts

1 package (10.5 ounces, or 300 g) cherry tomatoes, halved

½ cup (20 g) fresh chopped basil leaves

8 ounces (225 g) fresh mozzarella cheese balls, sliced

» Spray your crock with nonstick cooking spray.

» In a bowl, mix together the vinegar, oil, garlic, salt, and pepper. Arrange the chicken in the bottom of the crock and spread the tomatoes around the top. Pour the balsamic mixture over the chicken and tomatoes, top with the basil and finally, the cheese.

» Cover the crock and cook on LOW for 5 to 6 hours or on HIGH for 2½ to 3 hours.

RECOMMENDED SLOW COOKER SIZE:
5 quart (5 L) or larger

YIELD: 6 to 8 servings

TIPS & SUGGESTIONS

This pairs well with the Garlicky Veggie Medley on page 136 and the Mashed Cauliflower and Potatoes on page 142.

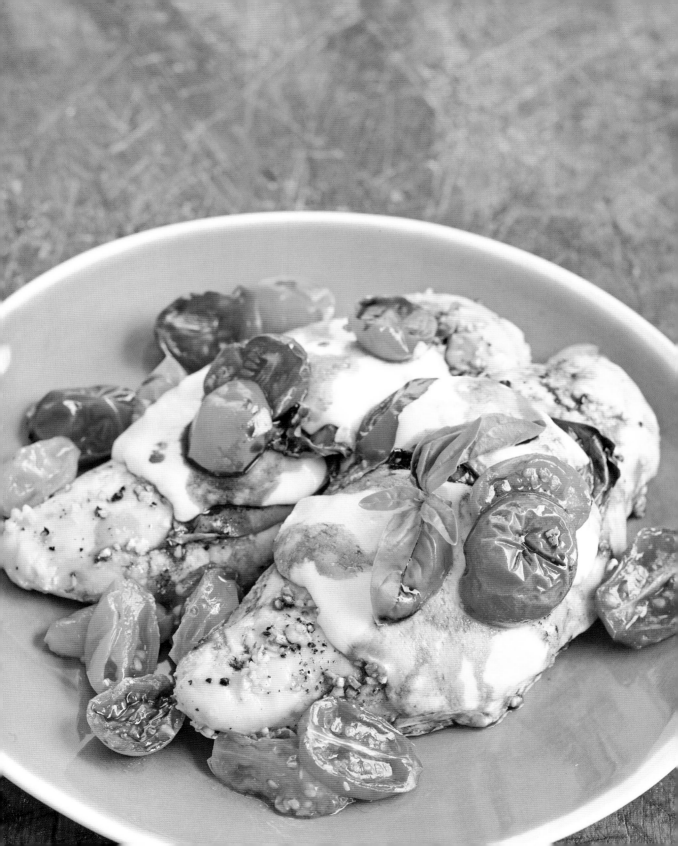

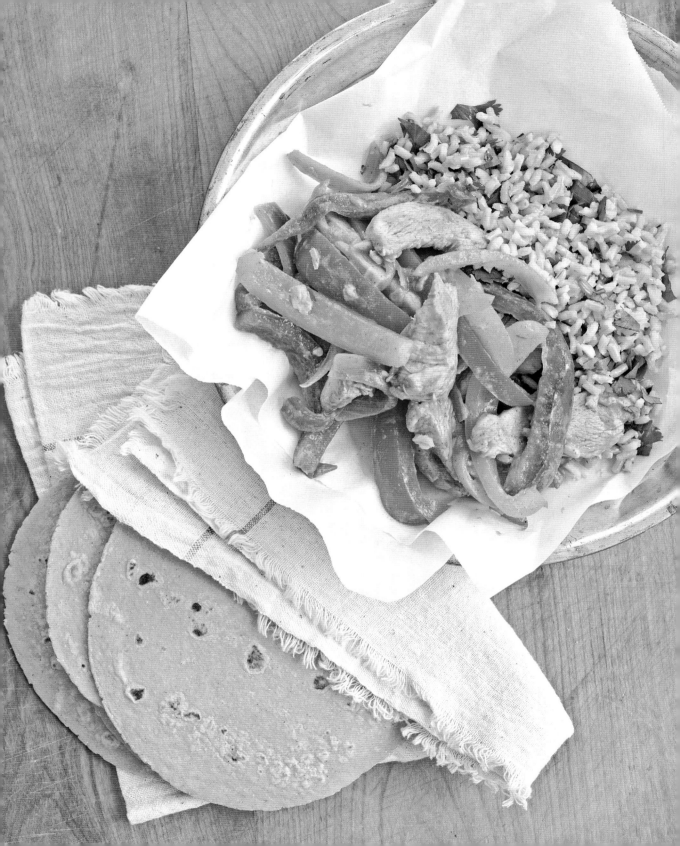

Chicken Fajitas

 5 INGREDIENTS OR LESS   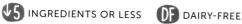 **DF** DAIRY-FREE

This recipe is quick and easy to throw together, and it only contains four ingredients. With just chicken, frozen veggies, taco seasoning, and cornstarch, you'll have a go-to meal for when you're in a real hurry.

3 pounds (1.4 kg) boneless, skinless chicken breasts, cut into 1½-inch (4 cm) strips

2 bags (16 ounces, or 455 g, total) frozen stir-fry vegetables

5 tablespoons (50 g) Taco Seasoning (page 72)

3 tablespoons (25 g) cornstarch

» Spray your crock with nonstick cooking spray.

» Place the chicken and vegetables into the crock. Sprinkle them with the taco seasoning and cornstarch, and then stir well.

» Cover the crock and cook on LOW for 5 to 6 hours or on HIGH for 2½ to 3 hours.

RECOMMENDED SLOW COOKER SIZE:
4 to 5 quart (4 to 5 L)

YIELD: 8 to 12 servings

 TIPS & SUGGESTIONS

» Serve this very simply over rice or on a gluten-free tortilla wrap, with or without rice.

» You can add any other vegetables you like, or use flank steak in place of the chicken.

Lime Chicken Tacos

 DAIRY-FREE

These tacos are simple and quick to throw together. The addition of lime in this recipe makes all of the difference. This is a huge hit in our house and a frequent request.

FOR THE CHICKEN:

1½ to 2 pounds (680 to 900 g) boneless, skinless chicken breasts

1 tablespoon (7 g) chili powder

2 limes, juiced

1 jar (16 ounces, or 455 g) salsa, divided

1 cup (130 g) frozen corn

SUGGESTED TOPPINGS:

Shredded lettuce

Chopped onion

Shredded cheese

Sour cream

Refried beans

Salsa or taco sauce

Black beans

» Spray your crock with nonstick cooking spray.

» Place the chicken into the crock.

» In a bowl, mix together the chili powder and lime juice and pour it over the top of the chicken along with half of the jar of salsa.

» Cover the crock and cook on LOW for 5 to 7 hours. (I do not recommend cooking this on HIGH.)

» Remove the chicken from the crock, shred it between two forks, and place it back into the crock. Pour the remaining salsa into the crock along with the frozen corn. Give it a stir.

» Cover the crock and cook for an additional ½ hour, or until everything is heated through.

» Serve with your choice of toppings.

RECOMMENDED SLOW COOKER SIZE:
3 quart (3 L)

YIELD: 4 to 6 servings

 TIPS & SUGGESTIONS

» Serve the chicken in crunchy taco shells, soft taco shells, or on top of tortilla chips for nachos instead.

» The chicken pairs well with the Butter and Herb Corn on the Cob on page 133 and some Spanish rice.

Chicken and Turkey Loaf

 DAIRY-FREE

Meatloaf is one of the simplest and most classic dinners out there. When I make it, I like to make a lot of it. I've been known to double this recipe just so I can have leftovers for more than one day. By using ground turkey and chicken, this meatloaf stays incredibly moist. It's seasoned with your favorite salsa and a couple of spices right out of your pantry. With this recipe, you'll have an incredibly flavorful dinner.

1 pound (455 g) ground turkey

1 pound (455 g) ground chicken

2 eggs, beaten

½ cup (130 g) salsa

1½ cups (175 g) gluten-free panko bread crumbs

1½ teaspoons dried minced onion

½ teaspoon cumin

½ teaspoon dried basil

» Spray your crock with nonstick cooking spray.

» In a large bowl, place the turkey, chicken, eggs, and salsa. Next, add the bread crumbs, onion, cumin, and basil. Using clean hands, mix the ingredients well. Form the meat mixture into a loaf and place it inside the crock.

» Cover the crock and cook on LOW for 5 to 6 hours or on HIGH for 2½ to 3 hours.

RECOMMENDED SLOW COOKER SIZE:
5 to 6 quart (5 to 6 L)

YIELD: 6 to 8 servings

 ## TIPS & SUGGESTIONS

Pair this with the Cheesy Broccoli Casserole on page 134, the Butter and Herb Corn on the Cob on page 133, and the Baked Sweet Potatoes on page 130.

Cranberry-Glazed Turkey Breast

DF DAIRY-FREE

Step out of your normal traditional comfort zone and try this spectacular glaze for your turkey breast. The sweetness of the cranberries mixed with the savory onion and other seasonings make this turkey breast superb.

1 turkey breast (5½ to 6 pounds, or 2.5 to 2.7 kg), giblets removed, rinsed, and dried

1 can (14 ounces, or 395 g) whole berry cranberry sauce

3 tablespoons (15 g) dried minced onion

1 teaspoon parsley flakes

1 teaspoon onion powder

1 teaspoon turmeric

1 teaspoon cornstarch

¼ teaspoon celery salt

¼ teaspoon granulated sugar

⅛ teaspoon ground black pepper

» Spray your crock with nonstick cooking spray.

» Place the turkey into the slow cooker, breast side down.

» In a bowl, mix together the cranberry sauce, onion, parsley, onion powder, turmeric, cornstarch, celery salt, sugar, and pepper. Pour the mixture all over the turkey breast.

» Cover the crock and cook on LOW for 8 to 9 hours or on HIGH for 4 to 4½ hours.

RECOMMENDED SLOW COOKER SIZE:
6½ to 7 quart (6½ to 7 L)

YIELD: 6 to 7 servings

 TIPS & SUGGESTIONS

This recipe pairs well with the Brown Sugar Mashed Sweet Potatoes on page 130, the Sweet Acorn Squash on page 135, the Honey-Lemon Glazed Carrots on page 142, and the Green Bean Casserole on page 139.

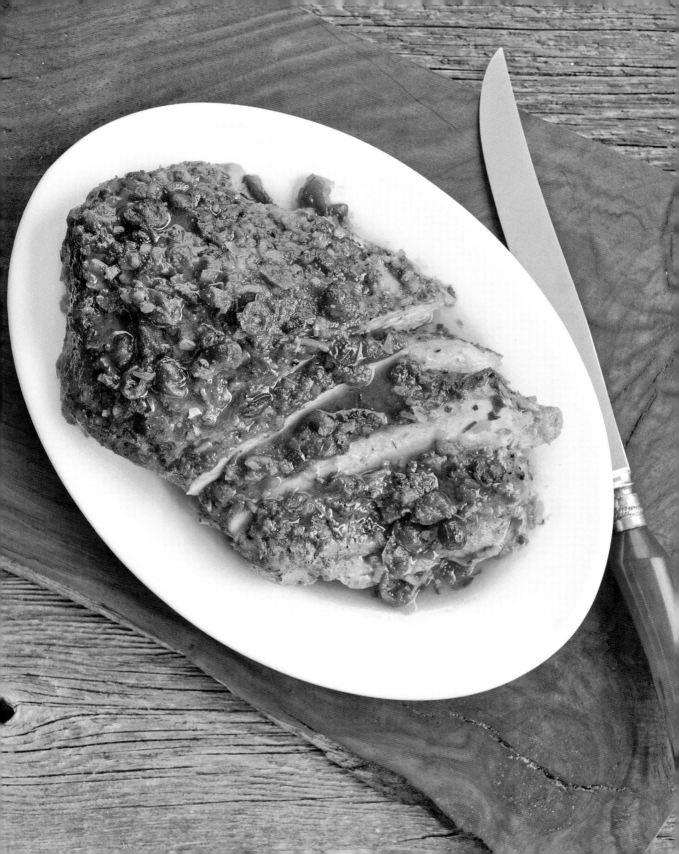

Garlic Chicken

 DAIRY-FREE

If you like a lot of garlic, you're going to *love* this chicken. These chicken breasts are covered with a delicious garlicky rub that create an incredible amount of flavor everyone will enjoy.

2 to 3 pounds (900 g to 1.4 kg) boneless, skinless chicken breasts
4 tablespoons (40 g) fresh minced garlic
1 teaspoon onion powder
1 tablespoon (14 ml) olive oil
1 teaspoon brown sugar
¼ teaspoon salt
⅛ teaspoon ground black pepper
2 tablespoons (28 ml) chicken stock

» Spray your crock with nonstick cooking spray.

» Place the chicken into the crock.

» In a bowl, mix together the garlic, onion powder, oil, sugar, salt, and pepper. Rub this all over the chicken in the crock. Pour in the stock.

» Cover the crock and cook on LOW for 5 hours or on HIGH for 2½ hours.

RECOMMENDED SLOW COOKER SIZE:
4 to 5 quart (4 to 5 L)

YIELD: 4 to 6 servings

TIPS & SUGGESTIONS

These are excellent served with the Garlic Mashed Sweet Potatoes on page 134 and the Garlicky Veggie Medley on page 136.

Herb-Crusted Pot Roast

 DAIRY-FREE

This is a great main dish for when you don't have time to hit the grocery store. Using herbs and spices you already have in your pantry, you can cook a delicious, tender, and incredibly flavorful roast.

FOR THE ROAST:
1 chuck or English roast (3 to 4 pounds, or 1.4 to 1.8 kg)
2 to 3 tablespoons (28 to 45 ml) olive oil

FOR THE RUB:
1 tablespoon (2 g) dried basil
1 tablespoon (3 g) dried oregano
1 tablespoon (1 g) dried parsley
2 teaspoons (6 g) garlic powder
1 teaspoon onion powder
1 teaspoon dried thyme
¼ teaspoon salt
¼ teaspoon ground black pepper

» Spray your crock with nonstick cooking spray.

» **To make the roast:** Place the roast into the crock and rub the oil all over it.

» **To make the rub:** In a small bowl, mix together all of the spices for the rub. Sprinkle this mixture over the roast, pressing it on the roast, turning the roast to make sure that all sides are coated.

» Cover the crock and cook on LOW for 8 to 10 hours or on HIGH for 4 to 5 hours.

RECOMMENDED SLOW COOKER SIZE:
3 to 5 quart (3 to 5 L)

YIELD: 6 servings

Herb-Stuffed Chicken

 DAIRY-FREE

"Simple and flavorful" is how I like to describe this chicken. By simply stuffing your chicken with a few fresh herbs and some garlic, this delicious chicken is an impressive dish to serve to your company.

1 whole chicken (3 to 4 pounds, or 1.4 to 1.8 kg), giblets removed, rinsed, and dried
6 whole garlic cloves
4 sprigs fresh thyme
3 to 4 sprigs fresh rosemary
1 sprig fresh sage
2 tablespoons (28 ml) olive oil
1 teaspoon sea salt
¼ teaspoon ground black pepper

Butcher's twine

» Ball up a few pieces of aluminum foil and place them on the bottom of your crock. (This will prop your chicken up out of the juices so it doesn't fall apart completely while it cooks.)

» Place the garlic inside the chicken. Tie together the thyme, rosemary, and sage with butcher's twine and stuff it inside the chicken, too. Truss the chicken with the butcher's twine.

Rub the chicken with the oil and sprinkle it with the salt and pepper. Place the chicken into the crock.

» Cover the crock and cook on LOW for 8 to 10 hours or on HIGH for 4 to 5 hours.

» Before serving, remove the chicken from the crock, un-truss it, and discard the butcher's twine. Remove the herbs from the chicken and discard them as well.

RECOMMENDED SLOW COOKER SIZE:
6 to 7 quart (6 to 7 L)

YIELD: 4 servings

RECIPE NOTE

Butcher's twine can sometimes be hard to find in grocery stores. You can ask at the meat counter, and they might even give you some for free! You can also look in the section of your grocery store where they sell kitchen utensils. Hardware stores and specialty cooking stores usually sell it as well.

TIPS & SUGGESTIONS

This recipe pairs well with the Sweet Acorn Squash on page 135, the Green Bean Casserole on page 139, and the Garlic Mashed Sweet Potatoes on page 134.

Honey Garlic Pork Chops

 INGREDIENTS OR LESS   **DAIRY-FREE**

Don't let the fact that this recipe has only five ingredients fool you. It's not boring. In fact, it's far from boring. Honey, garlic, salt, and pepper turn regular ole' pork chops into something *amazing*! This recipe pairs well with the Honey-Lemon Glazed Carrots on page 142, the Brown Sugar Mashed Sweet Potatoes on page 130, and the White Wine Mushrooms on page 135.

3 pounds (1.4 kg) pork chops
   (boneless or bone-in)
Salt, to taste
Ground black pepper, to taste
½ cup (170 g) honey
2 tablespoons (20 g) fresh, minced garlic

» Spray your crock with nonstick cooking spray.

» Place the pork into the crock and salt and pepper both sides.

» In a small bowl, mix together the honey and garlic. Pour the mixture over the pork.

» Cover the crock and cook on LOW for 7 to 8 hours or on HIGH for 3½ to 4 hours.

RECOMMENDED SLOW COOKER SIZE:
6 quart (6 L) or larger

YIELD: 4 to 6 servings

Jammin' Jerk Chicken

 INGREDIENTS OR LESS   **DAIRY-FREE**

With the first bite of this chicken, your senses will go into overdrive. Habanero peppers, mixed with a homemade sauce, create a spicy, sticky chicken that has lots of punch packed into each bite. This recipe pairs well with the Garlic Mashed Sweet Potatoes on page 134 and the Butter and Herb Corn on the Cob on page 133.

3 to 4 pounds (1.4 to 1.8 kg) bone-in chicken
   (Remove the skin if desired.)
2 habanero peppers, seeded and diced
1 tablespoon (15 ml) teriyaki sauce
1 teaspoon soy sauce
¼ cup (60 g) brown sugar
3 tablespoons (30 g) fresh minced garlic
1 teaspoon ginger
¼ teaspoon ground black pepper
½ teaspoon allspice

» Spray your crock with nonstick cooking spray.

» Place the chicken into the crock.

» In a bowl, mix together the remaining ingredients and pour the mixture over the chicken. Cover the crock and cook on LOW for 7 to 8 hours. (I do not recommend cooking this on HIGH.)

RECOMMENDED SLOW COOKER SIZE:
5 quart (5 L) or larger

YIELD: 6 servings

Kickin' Barbecue Shredded Beef

 INGREDIENTS OR LESS   DAIRY-FREE

Kickin' with spice and flavor, this shredded beef will not disappoint. With jalapeño slices and barbecue sauce, you turn a simple roast into a four-ingredient, amazingly tasty masterpiece.

1 boneless chuck roast (2½ to 3 pounds, or 1.1 to 1.4 kg)
1 cup (160 g) chopped red onion
1 jar (11.5 ounces, or 325 g) mild jalapeños
8 ounces (225 g) sweet barbecue sauce

» Spray your crock with nonstick cooking spray.

» Place the roast into the bottom of the crock and cover it with the onion. Pour the jalapeños, juice and all, over the top. Pour the barbecue sauce on top of that.

» Cover the crock and cook on LOW for 8 to 10 hours or on HIGH for 4 to 5 hours.

» Remove the roast from the crock and shred it with two forks, removing large pieces of fat as you go. Put the shredded beef back into the crock and stir it through the sauce.

RECOMMENDED SLOW COOKER SIZE:
3 to 5 quart (3 to 5 L)

YIELD: 8 to 10 servings

 TIPS & SUGGESTIONS

» This is delicious served traditionally on a gluten-free bun or roll.
» It would also be great in a lettuce wrap, over rice, on top of a gluten-free barbecue pizza, or on top of nachos.
» The beef pairs well with the Baked Sweet Potatoes on page 130.

MOUTHWATERING MAIN COURSES

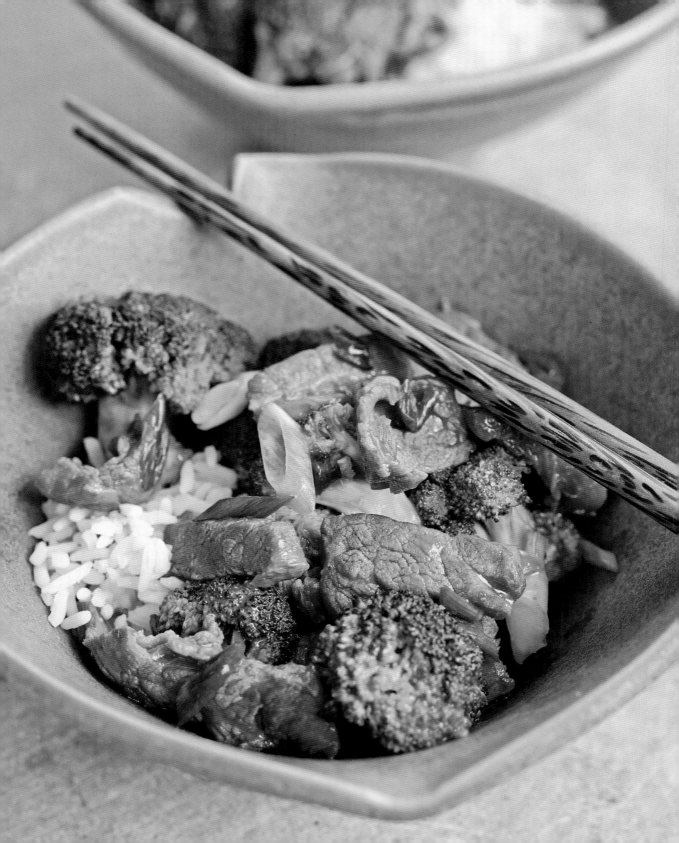

Mongolian Beef

 DAIRY-FREE

Having a hard time finding a Chinese place you can trust with your gluten-free needs? Don't bother calling! Save yourself the money and make this delicious Chinese-American dish at home. With flank steak, broccoli, scallions, and a few sauces and spices, you'll have a delicious "take-out" worthy meal.

1 pound (455 g) flank steak, cut into pieces (¼-inch [6 mm] thick × 1-inch [2.5 cm] wide)

16 ounces (455 g) frozen broccoli

4 scallions, sliced into 1-inch (2.5 cm) pieces

¼ cup (60 g) brown sugar

¼ cup (60 ml) soy sauce

1 teaspoon ginger

1 teaspoon fresh minced garlic

¼ cup (30 g) cornstarch

» Spray your crock with nonstick cooking spray.

» Place the steak, broccoli, and scallions into the crock.

» In a small bowl, mix together the sugar, soy sauce, ginger, and garlic. Slowly stir in the cornstarch. Pour the mixture over the steak and veggies and mix well.

» Cover the crock and cook on LOW for 4 hours or on HIGH for 2 hours.

RECOMMENDED SLOW COOKER SIZE:
2 quart (2 L)

YIELD: 4 servings

 ## TIPS & SUGGESTIONS

Serve this Mongolian Beef over white rice, brown rice, or quinoa. It pairs well with a nice salad as well.

Moroccan Chicken

 DAIRY-FREE

Want to serve your family or guests an "exotic" dinner that you don't have to run all over an exotic grocery store to make happen? You've come to the right place. This recipe offers all of the exotic flavors you want, with spices that you most likely already have in your pantry at home. This chicken is perfectly seasoned, and it will fall right off of the bone.

2 tablespoons (18 g) garlic powder

1 tablespoon (7 g) cumin

1 teaspoon turmeric

1 teaspoon paprika

1 teaspoon salt

½ teaspoon cinnamon

¼ teaspoon ground black pepper

¼ teaspoon coriander

4 pounds (1.8 kg) bone-in chicken, cuts of your choice

½ cup (120 ml) lemon juice

» Spray your crock with nonstick cooking spray.

» In a small bowl, mix together the garlic powder, cumin, turmeric, paprika, salt, cinnamon, pepper, and coriander.

» Place the chicken into the crock and sprinkle half of the seasoning mix you just made over that side of the chicken. Using tongs, turn the chicken over and sprinkle the remaining seasoning over the other side. Pour the lemon juice over the chicken.

» Cover the crock and cook on LOW for 8 hours of on HIGH for 4 hours.

RECOMMENDED SLOW COOKER SIZE:
6 quart (6 L) or larger

YIELD: 4 to 8 servings

 ## TIPS & SUGGESTIONS

This pairs well with Butter and Herb Corn on the Cob on page 133, White Wine Mushrooms on page 135, Herbed Fingerling Potatoes on page 140, Green Bean Casserole on page 139, Mashed Cauliflower and Potatoes on page 142, and Wild Rice with Veggies on page 146.

Paprika Chicken

 5 INGREDIENTS OR LESS 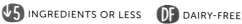 **DF DAIRY-FREE**

Save this recipe for a time when you're in a *huge* hurry. It literally takes minutes to throw together, but the results have a *huge* flavor! Smoked paprika, garlic, and diced tomatoes is all it takes to turn simple chicken into an amazing dinner.

4 pounds (1.8 kg) bone-in chicken, cuts of your choice

3 tablespoons (20 g) smoked paprika

1 tablespoon (10 g) fresh minced garlic

1 can (28 ounces, or 795 g) diced tomatoes

>> Spray your crock with nonstick cooking spray.

>> Place the chicken into the crock and sprinkle evenly with the paprika.

>> Mix the garlic into the can of tomatoes, and then pour the mixture over the chicken.

>> Cover the crock and cook on LOW for 8 hours or on HIGH for 4 hours.

RECOMMENDED SLOW COOKER SIZE:
6 to 7 quart (6 to 7 L)

YIELD: 6 to 8 servings

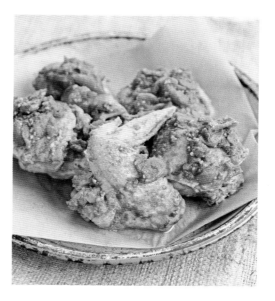

 ## TIPS & SUGGESTIONS

This chicken would be delicious alongside the Mashed Cauliflower and Potatoes on page 142, the Garlicky Veggie Medley on page 136, or even the Pizza-Stuffed Spaghetti Squash on page 145.

Perfect Hamburgers

I know you're reading this thinking, "Hamburgers? In a slow cooker?" I'm here to tell you that this is one of the best ways to cook your burgers. These come out so moist and flavorful. You'll love them, and your family and guests will love them, too.

¼ cup (60 ml) water

2 pounds (900 g) ground beef

1 egg, beaten

2 tablespoons (28 ml) Worcestershire sauce

1 package ranch dressing mix

1 tablespoon (5 g) dried minced onion

1½ teaspoons Italian seasoning

1 cup (115 g) gluten-free panko bread crumbs

» Crumple up several sheets of aluminum foil and place them on the bottom of your crock. (You're basically creating a platform for your burgers to sit on, but also a place for grease to drain so your burgers are not sitting in it.) Pour the water into the bottom of the crock.

» In a bowl, mix together the beef, egg, Worcestershire sauce, ranch dressing mix, onion, Italian seasoning, and bread crumbs. Form this mixture into 3-inch (7.5 cm) or so patties. Put 1 layer of burgers into your crock on top of the balls of foil.

» Take 3 pieces of foil and fold them into 1-inch (2.5 cm) wide strips. Lay these over the first layer of burgers in a star-shaped pattern. Lay your second layer of burgers on top. (This will keep your burgers from sticking together and allow the grease to continue to drain all of the way down.)

» Cover the crock and cook on LOW for 4 to 5 hours or on HIGH for 2 to 2½ hours.

RECOMMENDED SLOW COOKER SIZE:
5 to 6 quart (5 to 6 L)

YIELD: 7 to 8 servings

TIPS & SUGGESTIONS

» Instead of slaving over a grill at your next gathering, make these instead. They'll stay warm, and you'll be able to cook them all at once.

» These burgers pair well with the Pizza-Stuffed Spaghetti Squash on page 145 and the Butter and Herb Corn on the Cob on page 133.

RECIPE NOTE

To make this dairy-free, leave out the ranch dressing mix.

Spinach and Artichoke Chicken

Do you love chicken? Do you love spinach and artichoke dip? Then, you'll *love* this recipe. The creaminess of the cream cheese mixed with the fresh garlic creates an intense flavor, making this chicken dish a real crowd pleaser.

3 to 4 pounds (1.4 to 1.8 kg) boneless, skinless chicken breasts

1 can (15 ounces, or 425 g) artichoke hearts, drained and chopped

1 package (8 ounces, or 225 g) nonfat or reduced fat cream cheese, softened

8 ounces (225 g) frozen spinach, thawed, liquid squeezed out

½ cup (50 g) grated Parmesan cheese

2 tablespoons (20 g) fresh minced garlic

1 teaspoon salt

¼ teaspoon ground black pepper

» Spray your crock with nonstick cooking spray.

» Place the chicken into the bottom of the crock.

» In a bowl, mix together all of the remaining ingredients. Pour the mixture over the chicken.

» Cover and cook on LOW for 6 hours or on HIGH for 3 hours.

RECOMMENDED SLOW COOKER SIZE:
6 to 7 quart (6 to 7 L)

YIELD: 4 to 6 servings

TIPS & SUGGESTIONS

» Make this a complete meal by serving it with the Wild Rice with Veggies on page 146 and a fresh salad.

» This dish is wonderful served over quinoa or rice.

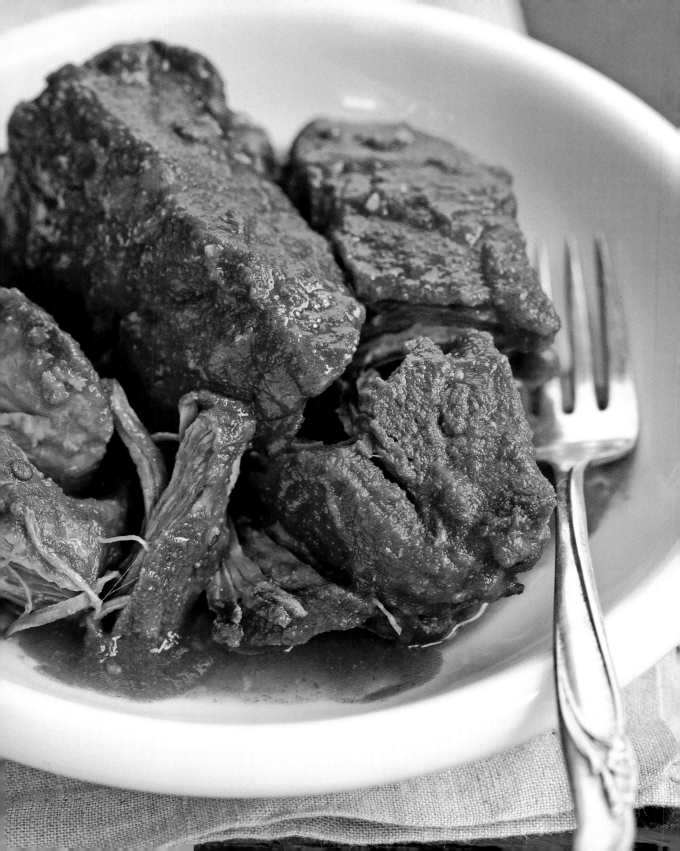

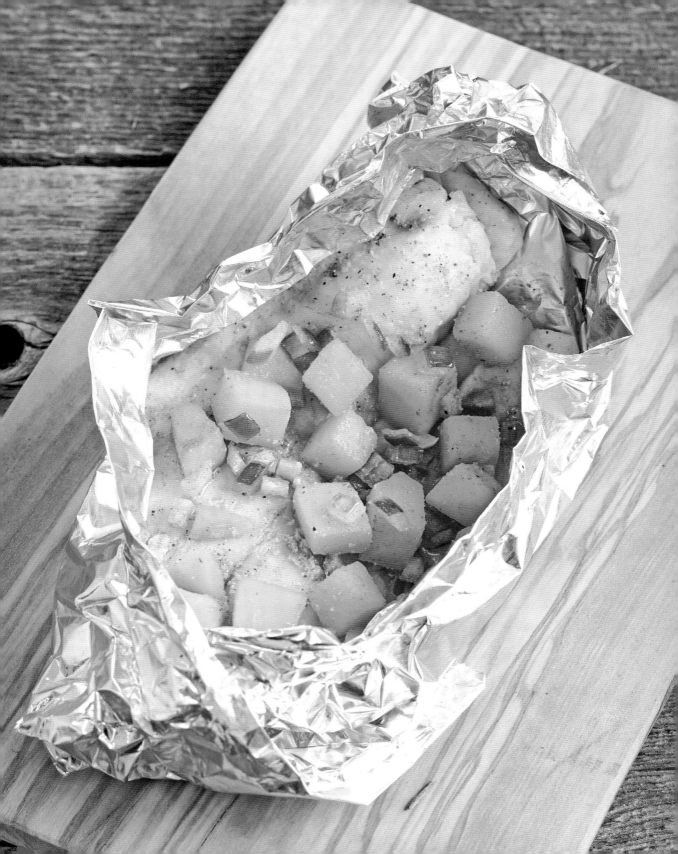

Garlic Butter–Poached Salmon

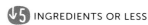 INGREDIENTS OR LESS

Butter, garlic, and salmon were meant to be together. By making this fish in simple foil packets, you won't have to worry about your fish falling apart when you turn it. After making this salmon in your slow cooker, you may never make it on the stove top again.

4 salmon filets (each 4 to 6 ounces,
   or 115 to 170 g)
4 teaspoons (12 g) garlic powder, divided
Salt, to taste
Ground black pepper, to taste
4 tablespoons (55 g) butter, divided

» On the counter, lay out four pieces of aluminum foil that are large enough to go beyond the length and width of your salmon filets by 3 to 4 inches (7.5 to 10 cm) in each direction. Place a salmon filet on each piece of aluminum foil.

» On each filet, sprinkle 1 teaspoon of the garlic powder, salt and pepper to taste, and 1 tablespoon (14 g) of the butter on top. Close up the packets and place them into your crock.

» Cover the crock and cook on LOW for 1 to 2 hours. (I do not recommend cooking this on HIGH.) The fish should flake easily with a fork when it is done.

RECOMMENDED SLOW COOKER SIZE:
4 to 5 quart (4 to 5 L)

YIELD: 4 servings

 TIPS & SUGGESTIONS

This dish pairs well with the Herbed Fingerling Potatoes on page 140 and the Garlicky Veggie Medley on page 136.

Eggplant Parmesan Casserole

There's no frying required in this simple, yet delicious, Eggplant Parmesan Casserole. The Italian seasoned bread crumbs, marinara sauce, and cheese make this a decadent, easy meal.

1 medium or 2 small eggplants

Salt

1 jar (8 ounces, or 225 g) marinara sauce, divided

1½ cups (175 g) gluten-free bread crumbs

1½ tablespoons (15 g) Italian seasoning

2 eggs or ½ cup (120 ml) egg whites

¾ cup (85 g) grated Parmesan cheese, divided

1 cup (115 g) shredded mozzarella cheese

Gluten-free pasta, for serving (optional)

» Spray your crock with nonstick cooking spray.

» Slice the eggplant into ½-inch (1 cm) thick rounds. Lay them on paper towel–lined baking sheets. Sprinkle both sides of each round with salt and allow the eggplant to "sweat" for at least 30 minutes. (Eggplant are full of moisture, so this prevents them from getting too soggy while cooking.) After 30 minutes, pat each piece of eggplant dry with paper towel.

» Pour about ¼ cup (60 g) marinara sauce into the bottom of the crock and spread it around.

» In a shallow bowl, mix together the bread crumbs and Italian seasoning.

» In another shallow bowl, beat the eggs or egg whites.

» Dredge each piece of eggplant in the eggs, coat each side with the bread crumbs, and then place it in the crock. Place enough eggplant slices to create one layer. Sprinkle the first layer with about one quarter of the Parmesan cheese and one-quarter of the marinara sauce. Repeat this process until you have about four layers.

» Cover the crock and cook on LOW for 5 to 6 hours or on HIGH for 2½ to 3 hours. The last ½ hour, sprinkle the mozzarella cheese on top and allow to melt. Serve as is or over gluten-free pasta.

RECOMMENDED SLOW COOKER SIZE:
3 quart (3 L)

YIELD: 6 servings

TIPS & SUGGESTIONS

» Serve this over some gluten-free pasta or quinoa.

» Conversely, if you're cutting down on carbs, serve this as is with a fresh salad or the White Wine Mushrooms on page 135.

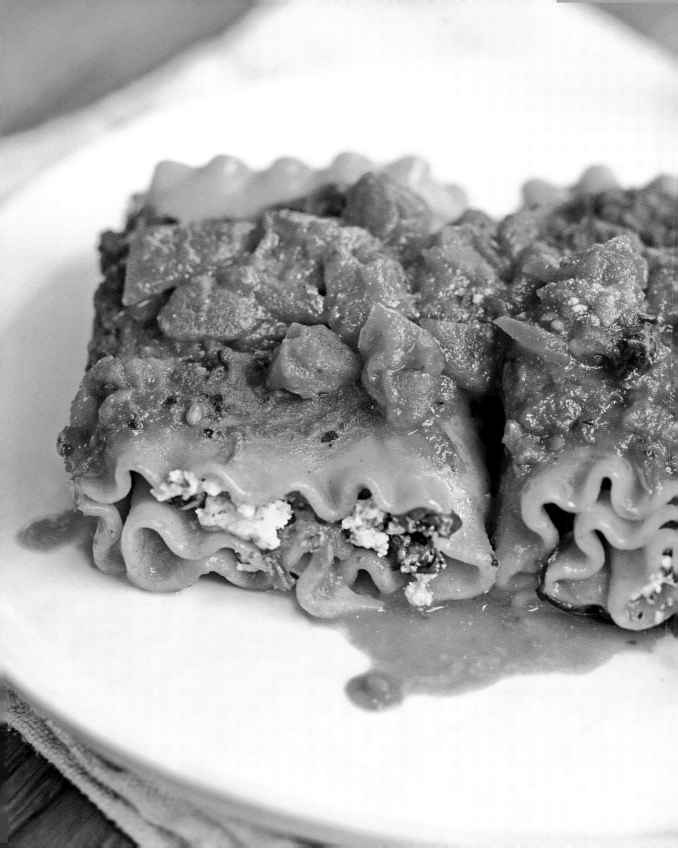

Lasagna Roll-Ups

✓5 INGREDIENTS OR LESS

When you want to change things up a little bit for dinner, might I suggest these lasagna roll-ups? With just lasagna noodles, ricotta cheese, fresh spinach, Italian seasoning, and marinara sauce, you'll have an impressive, unexpected dinner to put on the table.

1 package (10 ounces, or 280 g) gluten-free lasagna noodles

2 jars (24 ounces, or 680 g, each) marinara sauce, divided

15 ounces (425 g) ricotta cheese

1 tablespoon (10 g) Italian seasoning

1 cup (30 g) fresh spinach, divided

» Cook the noodles half of the time the instructions on the box say. Drain.

» Spray your crock with nonstick cooking spray. Pour about ½ cup (57 g) marinara sauce into the crock and spread it around.

» In a bowl, mix together the cheese and Italian seasoning.

» For each lasagna roll-up, lay a noodle on a clean surface and spread about 2 tablespoons (15 g) of the ricotta mixture across the entire length. Lay a few spinach leaves on top and spoon on about 1 tablespoon (7 g) of marinara sauce. Gently roll the lasagna noodles up and place the roll-ups into the crock. Place enough roll-ups to create one layer. Pour one-quarter of the marinara sauce on top of the first layer. Repeat to make two or three layers, finishing with marinara sauce on top.

» Cover and cook on LOW for 4 hours or on HIGH for 2 hours.

RECOMMENDED SLOW COOKER SIZE:
3 to 4 quart (3 to 4 L)

YIELD: 6 to 8 servings

TIPS & SUGGESTIONS

» Replace the spinach with beef.
» Add mozzarella cheese on top.
» Use cottage cheese instead of ricotta cheese.
» Pair with a green salad.

Lebanese Lentils and Rice (Mujadara)

 DAIRY-FREE

When I eat this dish, I automatically think of my childhood. My aunt would make Lebanese feasts for us monthly. This was just one of the many delicious dishes she made. When I was in college, I was always strapped for cash, so this was my go-to meal. It's incredibly inexpensive, and makes quite a bit. The sweetness of the caramelized onions is what really makes this dish spectacular. I always double this recipe because my husband can eat this for days on end.

½ cup (120 ml) olive oil

2 large sweet onions, roughly chopped

1 cup (190 g) uncooked lentils, rinsed

1 cup (190 g) uncooked brown rice

3 cups (700 ml) water

2 cups (475 ml) lemon juice

1 teaspoon salt

⅛ teaspoon ground black pepper

» Spray your crock with nonstick cooking spray.

» In a skillet, heat the oil. When the oil is hot, add the onion, coat it with the oil, and then turn the heat down to low. Cook the onion for about 1 hour, until it is brown and caramelized.

» Once the onions are caramelized, add the lentils and rice and coat them with the onion and oil. Add the mixture to your crock. Add the water, lemon juice, salt, and pepper to the crock and give it a quick stir.

» Cover the crock and cook on LOW for 8 hours or on HIGH for 4 hours.

RECOMMENDED SLOW COOKER SIZE:
3 quart (3 L)

YIELD: 6 servings

 TIPS & SUGGESTIONS

This dish is incredible in a lettuce wrap. You can also try this in a gluten-free soft tortilla shell, or you can be wild and crazy and eat it just as it is.

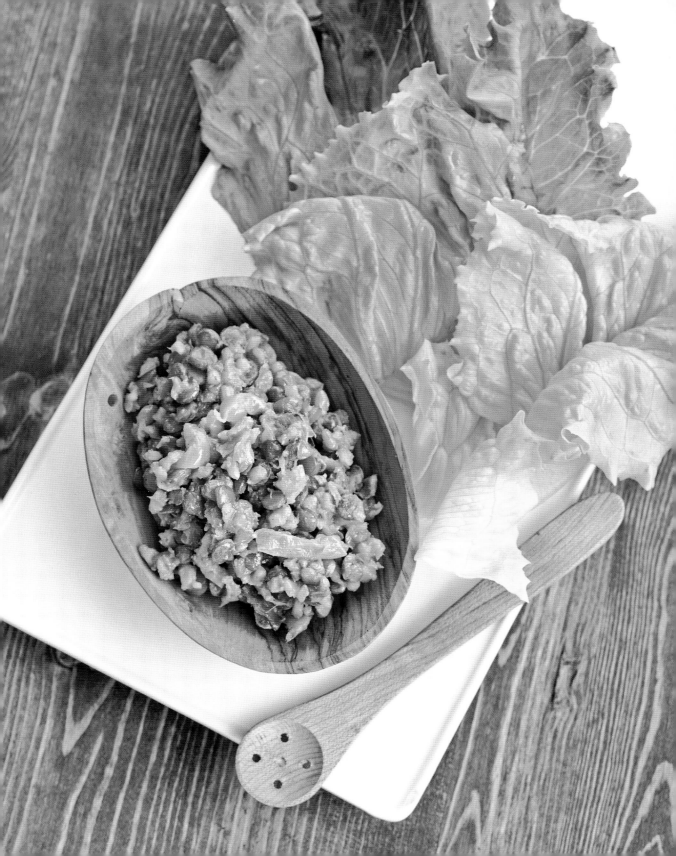

Lentil and Quinoa Tacos

DF DAIRY-FREE

Who knew that lentils and quinoa would make an awesome and immensely satisfying taco filling? This recipe is an incredibly flavorful alternative to traditional meat tacos. Your family won't miss the meat at all.

1 cup (190 g) uncooked lentils, rinsed

1 cup (175 g) uncooked quinoa, rinsed

6 cups (1.4 L) water

6 ounces (170 g) tomato paste

1 cup (160 g) chopped red onion

5 tablespoons (50 g) Taco Seasoning (page 72)

Soft or crunchy gluten-free taco shells, for serving

» Spray your crock with nonstick cooking spray.

» Place the lentils, quinoa, water, tomato paste, onion, and Taco Seasoning into the crock and stir.

» Cover the crock and cook on LOW for 8 hours or on HIGH for 4 hours.

» Serve the lentil and quinoa mixture on soft or crunch taco shells.

RECOMMENDED SLOW COOKER SIZE:
6 quart (6 L) or larger

YIELD: 8 to 12 servings

TIPS & SUGGESTIONS

» Serve these with soft or crunchy gluten-free yellow corn tortillas.

» Top with all of your favorite extras, such as shredded cheese, sour cream, plain Greek yogurt, onions, tomatoes, lettuce, and taco sauce.

Vegetarian Stuffed Peppers

Bring your tastebuds to life with these delicious stuffed peppers. With two kinds of beans, fresh tomatoes, parsley, spinach, some common spices, and a jar of marinara sauce, these stuffed peppers will wow your family or your company.

2 cups (330 g) cooked brown rice

½ can (15.5 ounces, or 440 g) black beans, rinsed and drained

½ can (15.5 ounces, or 440 g) cannelloni beans, rinsed and drained

1 large heirloom tomato, chopped

3 cups (90 g) fresh spinach

¼ cup (15 g) chopped fresh parsley

1½ cups (175 g) shredded mozzarella cheese (omit for dairy-free)

2 teaspoons (6 g) garlic powder

2 teaspoons (5 g) onion powder

1 teaspoon salt

6 bell peppers, tops removed and seeded (colors of your choosing)

1 jar (24 ounces, or 680 g) marinara sauce

½ teaspoon ground black pepper

» Spray your crock with nonstick cooking spray.

» In a bowl, mix together the rice, black beans, cannelloni beans, tomato, spinach, parsley, cheese, garlic powder, onion powder, salt, and black pepper.

» Evenly divide the rice mixture between the bell peppers, really packing the mixture into the peppers tightly. Place the peppers into the slow cooker. Pour the marinara sauce over the top of the peppers.

» Cover the crock and cook on LOW for 6 hours or on HIGH for 3 hours.

RECOMMENDED SLOW COOKER SIZE:
6 quart (6 L) or larger

YIELD: 6 servings

TIPS & SUGGESTIONS

This dish pairs well with a salad.

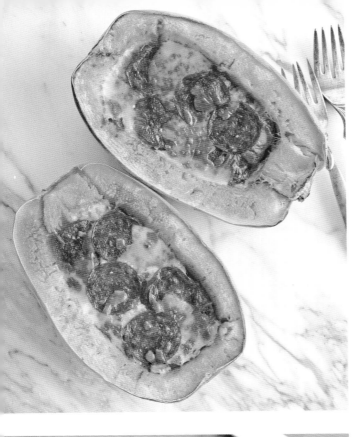
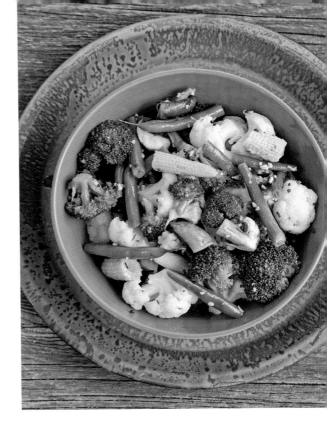
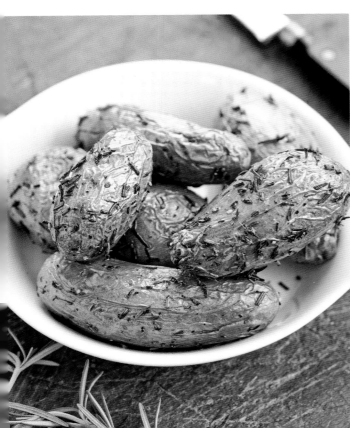
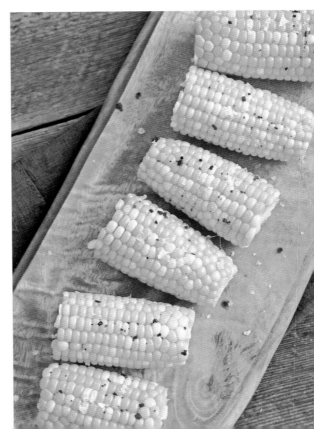

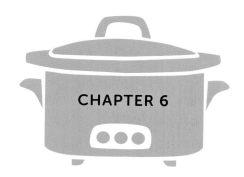

CHAPTER 6

SCRUMPTIOUS SIDE DISHES

Your slow cooker isn't just good for the main course. Oh no! It's great for your side dishes as well. Whether you're asked to bring a side dish to a family gathering or work party, you're hosting a party, or you're just having dinner at home, you're sure to find the perfect recipe in this chapter.

Baked Sweet Potatoes

 INGREDIENTS OR LESS   DAIRY-FREE

Having naturally sweet and delicious sweet potatoes with your dinner just got a whole lot easier. Simply poke your potatoes, put them in your slow cooker, and walk away! That's it. Come dinner time, you'll have a healthy side dish to serve with your main course.

6 to 8 sweet potatoes

» Spray your crock with nonstick cooking spray.

» Wash and dry each sweet potato and poke them all over with a knife or fork. Place them into your crock.

» Cover the crock and cook on LOW for 4 to 5 hours, or until the potatoes are tender. (I do not recommend cooking this on HIGH.)

RECOMMENDED SLOW COOKER SIZE:
6 quart (6 L) or larger

YIELD: 6 to 12 servings

Brown Sugar Mashed Sweet Potatoes

 INGREDIENTS OR LESS

This recipe provides all the goodness of mashed potatoes, but it's sweet and delicious instead of savory. You won't need dessert after eating these amazingly easy sweet potatoes.

6 cups (660 g) ½-inch (1 cm) peeled sweet potato cubes
⅓ cup (75 g) brown sugar
6 tablespoons (85 g) butter
½ cup (120 ml) vegetable stock

» Spray your crock with nonstick cooking spray.

» Place the sweet potatoes into the crock and sprinkle the sugar over the top. Place the butter on top, and then pour the stock over the top as well.

» Cover the crock and cook on LOW for 6 hours or on HIGH for 3 hours, or until the potatoes are very tender and pierce easily with a fork. Mash the potatoes right in the crock.

RECOMMENDED SLOW COOKER SIZE:
2 to 3 quart (2 to 3 L)

YIELD: 6 to 8 servings

TIPS & SUGGESTIONS

This dish pairs well with the Chicken and Turkey Loaf on page 101 and the Kickin' Barbecue Shredded Beef on page 107.

TIPS & SUGGESTIONS

This dish pairs well with the Apple and Onion Pork Loin on page 92, the Cranberry-Glazed Turkey Breast on page 102, and the Honey Garlic Pork Chops on page 106.

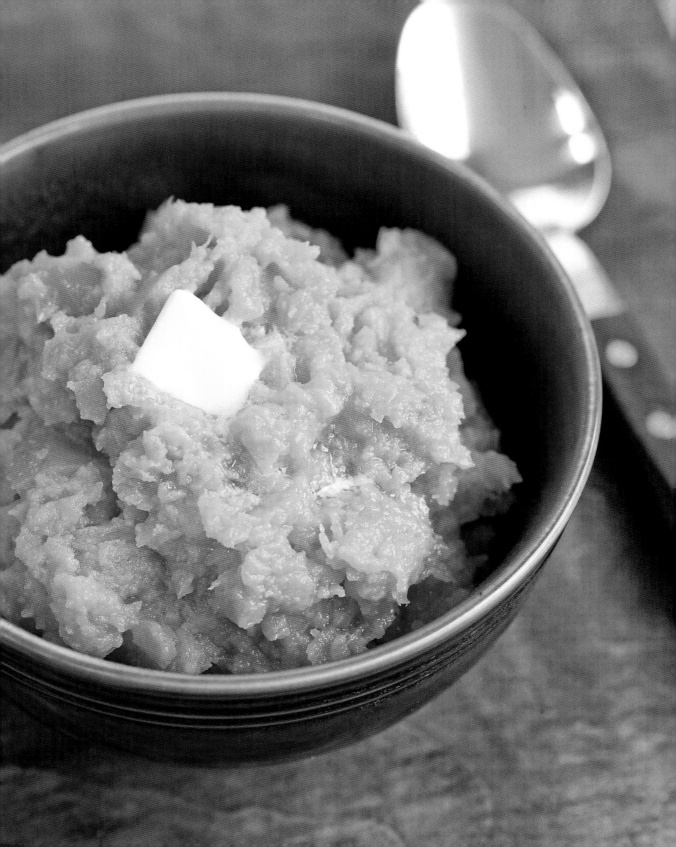

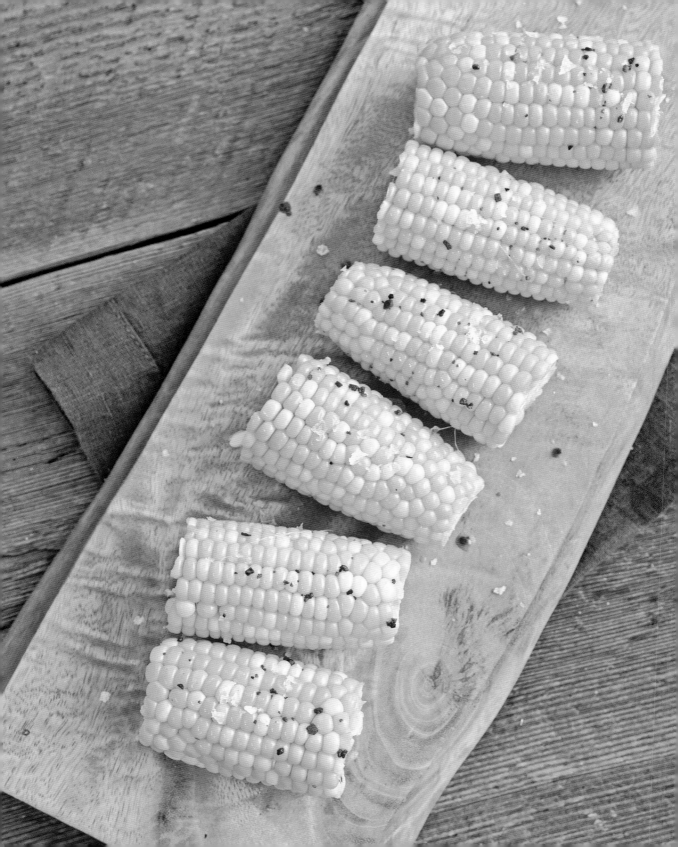

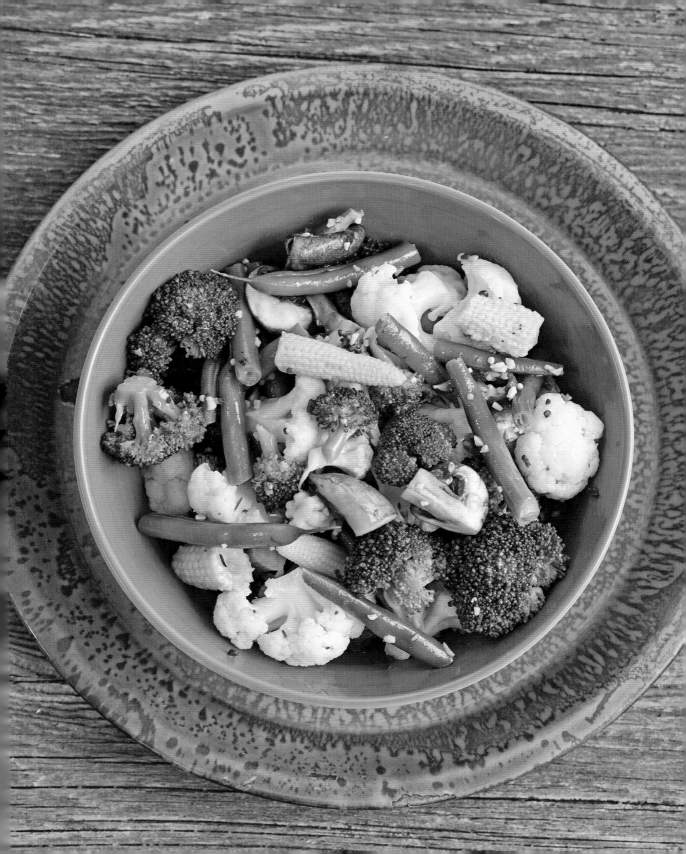

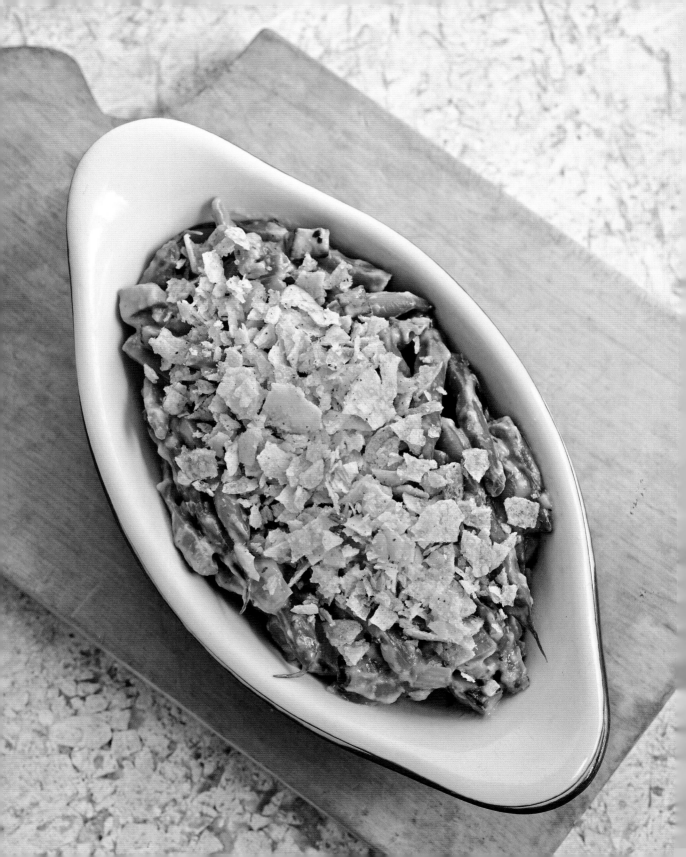

Green Bean Casserole

This is a lighter version of the traditional green bean casserole with the French-fried onions you may be used to. Using homemade cream of mushroom soup, you'll cut down on the calories and sodium you would normally consume by using canned, condensed soup. By using fresh green beans in this recipe, you'll still be able keep the slight crispiness of the green bean intact.

FOR THE GREEN BEANS:

4 pounds (1.8 kg) fresh green beans, cut bite-size and ends snipped

½ cup (80 g) diced onion

½ cup (30 g) crushed sour cream and onion potato chips

FOR THE SOUP:

1 teaspoon olive oil

3 mushrooms, diced

2 cups (475 ml) vegetable or chicken stock

⅔ cups (85 g) dry milk powder

¾ teaspoon garlic powder

¾ teaspoon onion powder

¾ teaspoon dried minced onion

¼ teaspoon salt

⅛ teaspoon dried basil

⅛ teaspoon dried parsley

⅛ teaspoon ground black pepper

⅓ cup (40 g) cornstarch

» Spray your crock with nonstick cooking spray.

» To make the green beans: Place the green beans and onion into the crock.

» To make the soup: In a sauce pan, heat the oil over medium-high. Place the mushrooms into the heated oil and cook them until they are soft. Add in the stock along with the dry milk powder, garlic powder, onion powder, onion, salt, basil, parsley, and pepper. Using a whisk, slowly whisk in the cornstarch little by little. Whisk constantly until everything is smooth. Allow the liquid to come to a low boil until it is thickened appropriately to the consistency of cream of mushroom soup.

» Pour the over the green beans and onions and mix it around.

» Cover the crock and cook on LOW for 4 to 5 hours or on HIGH for 2 to 2½ hours.

» When the cook time is over and the green beans are cooked, stir them and sprinkle the potato chips over the top.

RECOMMENDED SLOW COOKER SIZE:
2½ quart (2½ L)

YIELD: 8 to 10 servings

 ## TIPS & SUGGESTIONS

This dish pairs well with the Cranberry-Glazed Turkey Breast on page 102 or the Herb-Stuffed Chicken on page 105.

Herbed Fingerling Potatoes

 DAIRY-FREE

Coated with some olive oil, fresh thyme, rosemary, basil, salt, and pepper, these fingerling potatoes will melt in your mouth. Even though this recipe doesn't qualify as five ingredients or less, it's still super simple, with only seven ingredients.

24 ounces (680 g) fingerling potatoes
2 tablespoons (28 ml) olive oil
1 tablespoon (2 g) minced fresh thyme
1 tablespoon (2 g) rosemary
1 teaspoon dried basil
1 teaspoon sea salt
⅛ teaspoon ground black pepper

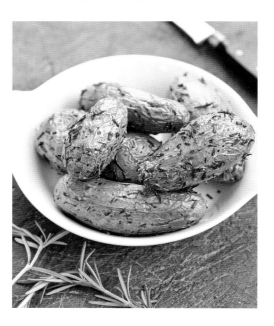

» Spray your crock with nonstick cooking spray.

» Place the potatoes into the crock and pour the oil over the top. Add the thyme, rosemary, basil, salt, and pepper into your crock. Mix up everything well so that the potatoes are well coated with the oil and spices.

» Cover the crock and cook on LOW for 5 to 6 hours or on HIGH for 2½ to 3 hours.

RECOMMENDED SLOW COOKER SIZE:
2 to 3 quart (2 to 3 L)

YIELD: 6 to 8 servings

 ## TIPS & SUGGESTIONS

This dish pairs well with the Herb-Crusted Pot Roast on page 104, the Tangy Barbecue Pulled Pork on page 116, and the Garlic Butter–Poached Salmon on page 120.

Kickin' Warm Bean Salad

With just a few simple and healthy ingredients, you can make this kickin' warm bean salad to accompany your dinner or to bring to a family gathering or picnic. Jazzing up dinnertime has never been so easy.

1 can (15.5 ounces, or 440 g) Great Northern Beans, rinsed and drained

1 can (15.5 ounces, or 440 g) black beans, rinsed and drained

¾ cup (170 g) chopped tomato

1 banana pepper, seeded and minced

1 tablespoon olive oil

1 tablespoon lemon juice

2 teaspoons (6 g) fresh, minced garlic

Salt and pepper, to taste

» Place the Great Northern beans, black beans, tomato, and banana pepper into the crock. Add in the olive oil, lemon juice, minced garlic, salt, and pepper. Give it a quick stir.

» Cook on LOW for 4 to 6 hours or on HIGH for 2 to 3 hours.

RECOMMENDED SLOW COOKER SIZE:
1½ to 2 quarts (1½ to 2 L)

YIELD: 6 to 8 servings

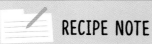

RECIPE NOTE

This side dish pairs well with Zesty Pork Burritos on page 117, Sweet and Spicy Chipotle Boneless Country Ribs on page 115, and Perfect Hamburgers on page 112.

Mashed Cauliflower and Potatoes

If you don't tell your guests, they will never know there is cauliflower in these mashed potatoes. The cauliflower brings a depth of flavor to these simple mashed potatoes that is incredible. With no water to boil and no potatoes to drain, these simple mashed cauliflower and potatoes are super easy to make.

3 pounds (1.4 kg) Idaho potatoes, cut into ½-inch (1 cm) cubes
2 cups (260 g) frozen cauliflower
½ cup (120 ml) vegetable stock
5 tablespoons (70 g) butter, divided into 5 pieces
½ teaspoon salt
¼ teaspoon ground black pepper
¼ cup (60 ml) milk
¾ cup (175 g) nonfat plain Greek yogurt

» Spray your crock with nonstick cooking spray.

» Place the potatoes into the crock, topped with the cauliflower. Pour in the stock and top it with the butter.

» Cover the crock and cook on LOW for 7 to 8 hours, or until the potatoes are tender. (Test them with a fork. I do not recommend trying to cook this on HIGH.)

» Add the salt, pepper, milk, and yogurt, and then mash the potatoes with a potato smasher right in the crock. (Don't overmix the potatoes, or they will become "gluey." Just mash/mix them until everything is combined and mashed pretty well. It's okay to have little chunks in there.)

RECOMMENDED SLOW COOKER SIZE:
3 to 4 quart (3 to 4 L)

YIELD: 8 to 10 servings

Honey-Lemon Glazed Carrots

 INGREDIENTS OR LESS

You will probably never prepare carrots any other way after tasting these delicious little beauties. These carrots are so sweet and delicious that they're almost like dessert. These will quickly become one of your family favorite recipes.

1 bag (32 ounces, or 1 kg) baby carrots
½ cup (170 g) honey
3 tablespoons (45 g) butter, melted
¼ cup (60 ml) lemon juice
1½ tablespoons (6 g) fresh minced parsley

» Spray your crock with nonstick cooking spray.

» Place the carrots into your crock and pour in the honey, butter, and lemon juice. Mix it around.

» Cover the crock and cook on LOW for 8 hours or on HIGH for 4 hours.

» When the cook time is up and the carrots are cooked, sprinkle in the parsley before serving.

RECOMMENDED SLOW COOKER SIZE:
2½ to 3 quart (2½ to 3 L)

YIELD: 8 to 10 servings

 TIPS & SUGGESTIONS

This dish pairs well with the Cranberry-Glazed Turkey Breast on page 102, the Honey Garlic Pork Chops on page 106, the Moroccan Chicken on page 110, and the Mango Salsa Tilapia on page 118.

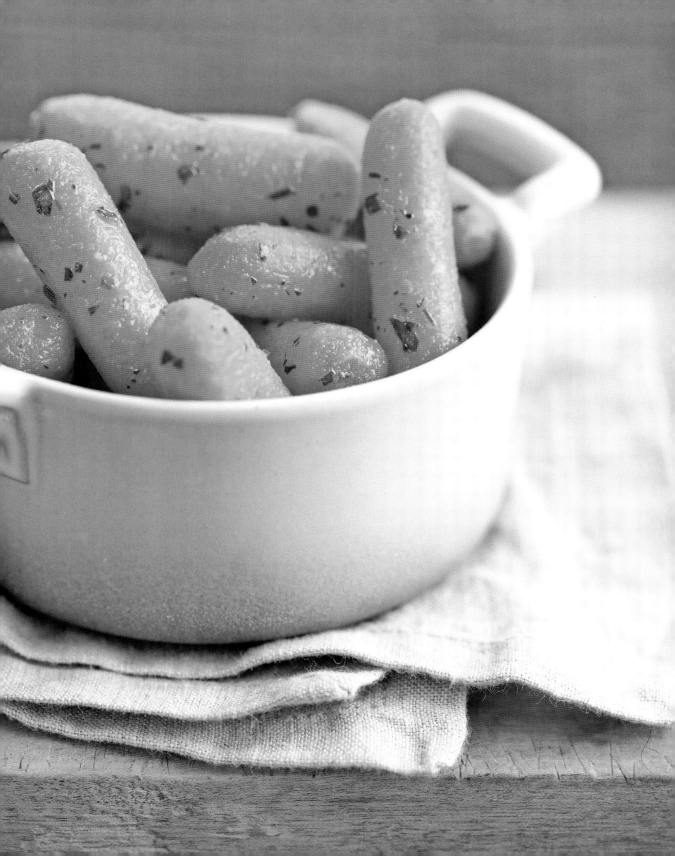

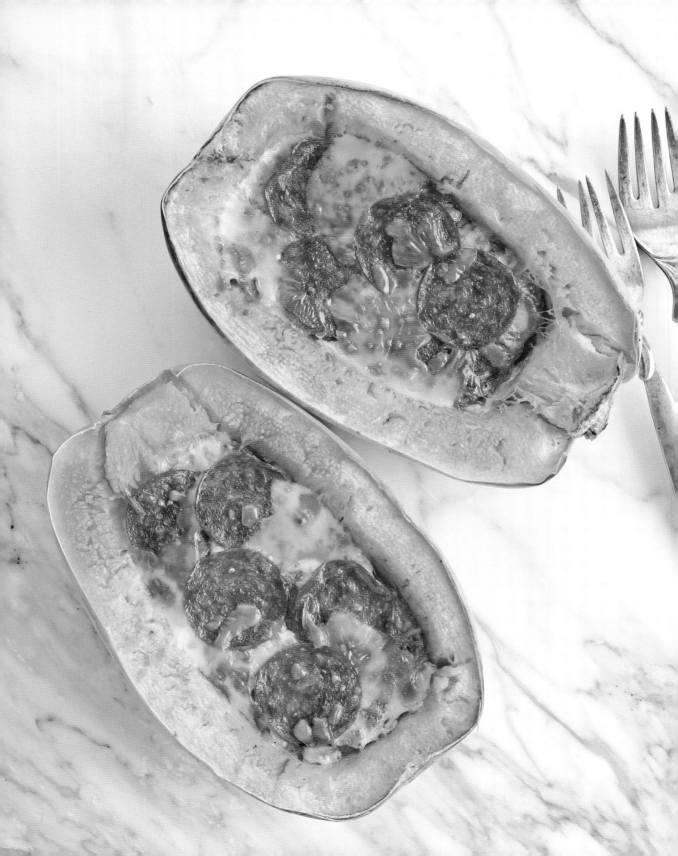

Pizza-Stuffed Spaghetti Squash

These little boats of pizza goodness are a fun way to spice up your usual dinner "sides." With all of the tastiness of pizza, but with the healthier twist of spaghetti squash, your family will fall in love with this super-creative side dish.

1 medium to large spaghetti squash
15 ounces (425 g) pizza sauce
¼ cup (35 g) grated Parmesan cheese
¼ cup (30 g) gluten-free bread crumbs
⅓ cup (30 g) turkey pepperoni, diced,
   plus 12 to 16 whole pieces
½ cup (60 g) shredded mozzarella, divided

» Spray your crock with nonstick cooking spray.

» Cut the spaghetti squash in half and scrape out the seeds and pulp. Place the squash halves into your slow cooker(s).

» In a bowl, mix together the pizza sauce with the Parmesan cheese, bread crumbs, and diced pepperoni. Gently pour the mixture evenly into both squash halves. Top each half with the whole pieces of pepperoni and the mozzarella cheese.

» Cover the crock and cook on LOW for 4 hours or on HIGH for 2 hours. When it's time to serve, gently scrape the squash with a fork to make it "spaghetti" up for you.

RECOMMENDED SLOW COOKER SIZE:
5 to 7 quart (5 to 7 L) Note: You may need to use two slow cookers—one for each half of squash, depending on the size and shape of the squash that you choose.

YIELD: 6 servings

TIPS & SUGGESTIONS

This dish pairs well with the Paprika Chicken on page 111 and the Perfect Hamburgers on page 112.

Wild Rice with Veggies

 DAIRY-FREE

Free up your stove top by cooking this delicious side in your slow cooker instead. With the addition of lots of veggies, this rice becomes a super healthy side dish. It would make an excellent accompaniment to almost any meal.

1 cup (160 g) uncooked wild rice

½ cup (65 g) chopped carrots

½ cup (65 g) frozen peas

¼ cup (40 g) diced red pepper

½ cup (35 g) diced mushrooms

¼ cup (40 g) chopped onion

½ teaspoon salt

⅛ teaspoon ground black pepper

1 teaspoon seasoning blend, such as Mrs. Dash Original Seasoning

1 teaspoon garlic powder

3 cups (700 ml) chicken stock (or vegetable stock if you want this to be vegetarian)

2 tablespoons (8 g) fresh minced parsley

» Spray your crock with nonstick cooking spray.

» Place the rice, carrots, peas, red pepper, mushrooms, onion, salt, black pepper, seasoning blend, and garlic powder into the crock. Pour the stock over the top.

» Cover the crock and cook on LOW for 3 to 4 hours, or until the rice and vegetables reach the desired tenderness. (I do not recommend cooking this on HIGH.)

» When you're ready to serve this rice, toss it with the parsley.

RECOMMENDED SLOW COOKER SIZE:
2 to 3 quart (2 to 3 L)

YIELD: 4 to 6 servings

 TIPS & SUGGESTIONS

This dish pairs well with the Herb-Crusted Pot Roast on page 104 and the Spinach and Artichoke Chicken on page 113.

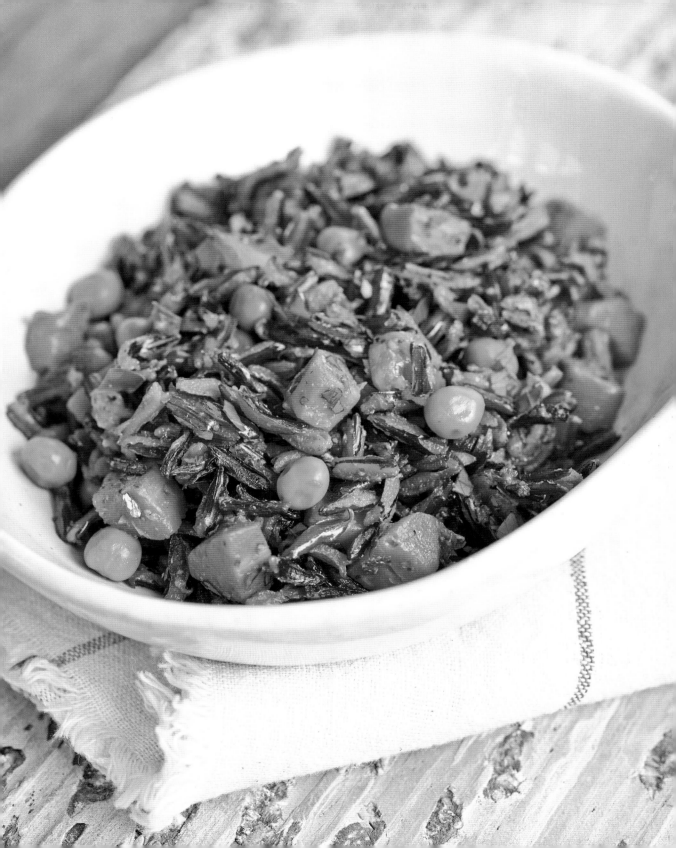

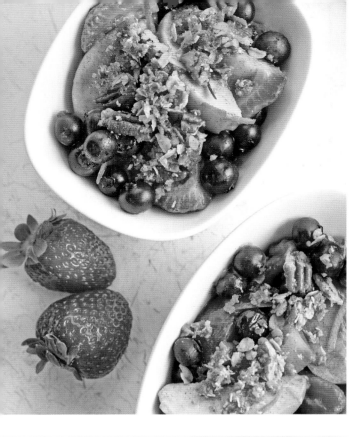

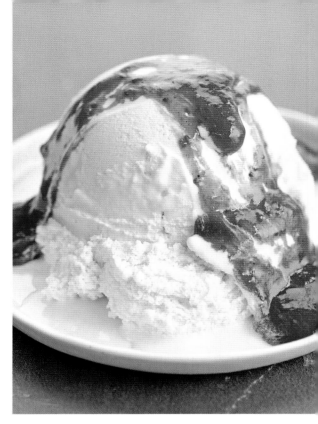

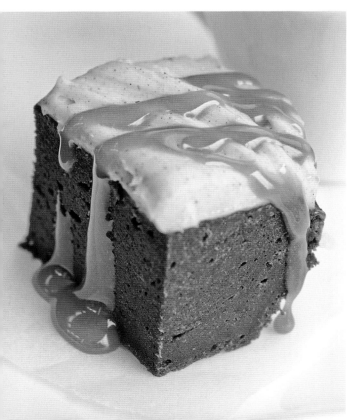

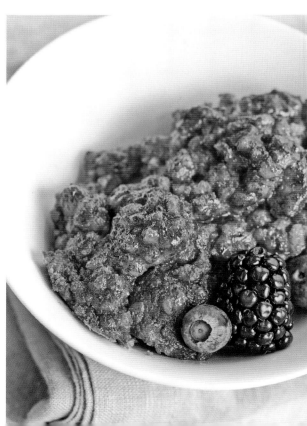

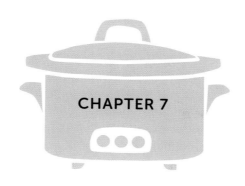

CHAPTER 7

DREAMY DESSERTS

Why take up precious oven space or heat up your kitchen for dessert when you can use your slow cooker instead? In this chapter, you'll find cakes, brownies, cobblers, puddings, and more. There's something for everyone and recipes I hope you'll make for years to come.

Coffee Caramel Cake

When you put the words "coffee, caramel, and cake" into the same sentence, you know it's going to be good. This cake has an incredible coffee flavor and even more dreaminess with the addition of a coffee-flavored frosting, drizzled with incredible caramel sauce.

FOR THE CAKE:

1 box (22 ounces, or 625 g) gluten-free yellow or white cake mix, plus the ingredients it calls for

2 tablespoons (10 g) instant coffee

¾ cup (175 ml) Caramel Sauce (page 165), divided

FOR THE FROSTING:

1 stick (110 g) butter, softened

5 tablespoons (65 g) vegetable shortening

1 teaspoon vanilla

⅔ cup (155 ml) milk, room temperature

1 teaspoon instant coffee

1 cup (200 g) granulated sugar

» To make the cake: Line your crock with parchment paper, and then spray well with nonstick cooking spray. Prepare the cake mix according to the package directions, and then add in the instant coffee. Pour the batter into the crock and drizzle it with ½ cup (120 ml) of the Caramel Sauce.

» Cover the crock and cook on LOW for 3 to 4 hours, depending on the size and shape of your crock, or until a toothpick comes out of the center clean. (I do not recommend cooking this on HIGH.) Remove the cake from the crock by pulling up on the parchment paper edges and place it on a cooling rack.

» To make the frosting: When the cake is almost cool, make the frosting. In a bowl, using an electric mixer, beat together the butter, shortening, and vanilla until it is smooth.

» In another bowl, mix together the milk and the instant coffee until the coffee is dissolved.

» Alternately pour the milk/coffee mixture and the sugar into the butter/vegetable shortening/vanilla mixture as you continue to beat it on a low speed. Once it's well combined, continue to beat it on a higher speed for about 10 minutes. (It should be completely smooth.)

Frost your cake once it's completely cooled and drizzle each piece with the reserved Caramel Sauce when serving.

RECOMMENDED SLOW COOKER SIZE:
6 to 7 quart (6 to 7 L)

YIELD: 12 to 15 servings

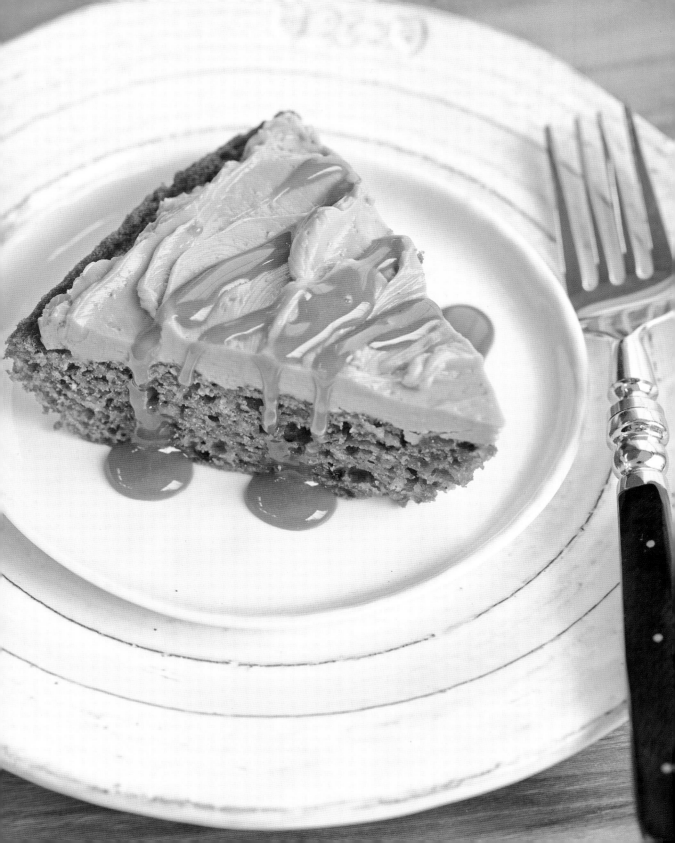

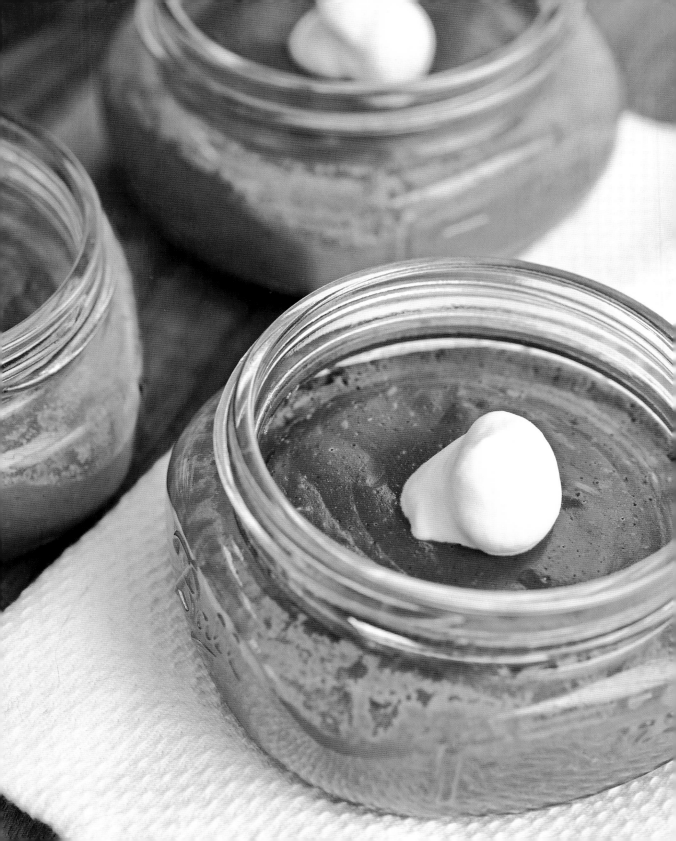

Hazelnut and Chocolate Mini Cheesecakes

These individual cheesecakes are decadent, smooth, creamy, hazelnutty, chocolaty, and delicious. They are incredibly charming, served in individual mason jars, which makes for a beautiful presentation for your guests.

1 box (8 ounces, or 225 g) reduced-fat cream cheese, softened

1 cup (230 g) nonfat plain Greek yogurt

⅓ cup (60 g) granulated sugar

1 teaspoon vanilla

2 eggs

¾ cup (195 g) chocolate-hazelnut spread, such as Nutella

6 mason jars (6 ounces, or 175 ml, each)

» Using a stand mixer, beat together the cream cheese, yogurt, sugar, and vanilla on medium-low speed. (You may use a hand mixer if you do not have a stand mixer.) When it is well mixed, add the eggs, one at a time. When this is well combined, add the chocolate-hazelnut spread. Continue to mix and scrape the sides of the bowl as necessary.

» When the mixture is well combined, pour or spoon the batter evenly into the 6 jars. Leaving the lid off of the jars, place them into your crock. Carefully pour water into the crock around the outside of the jars, until the water level is about halfway up the outside of the mason jars. (Be careful not to get any water in your cheesecakes.)

» Cover the crock and cook on LOW for 4 to 5 hours or on HIGH for 2 to 2½ hours.

» When the cook time is up, wearing an oven mitt, *carefully* remove the mason jars from the water bath and place them on a cooling rack.

RECOMMENDED SLOW COOKER SIZE:
5 quart (5 L) or larger

YIELD: 6 servings

TIPS & SUGGESTIONS

» Tie a ribbon around each jar, correlating to whatever theme or holiday you're celebrating.

» For serving, top each cheesecake with a dollop of whipped cream and some mini chocolate chips.

Chocolate Lava Cake

The chocolate fudge pudding is the secret to making this chocolate lava cake one of the best you will ever taste. It's gooey, chocolaty, and delicious!

1 box (22 ounces, or 625 g) gluten-free chocolate cake mix, plus the ingredients it calls for
1½ cups (265 g) milk chocolate chips
1 box (3.9 ounces, or 110 g) instant chocolate fudge pudding, plus the ingredients it calls for

» Line your crock with parchment paper and spray well with nonstick cooking spray.

» Prepare the cake mix according to the directions on the box and pour it into the crock. Sprinkle the chocolate chips all over the top.

» Prepare the chocolate pudding according to the directions on the box and pour it over the middle of the cake mix.

» Cover the crock and cook on LOW for 5 hours or on HIGH for 2½ hours, or until the sides have puffed up and are spongy and feel "done." (The middle will not set. It stays nice and gooey!)

RECOMMENDED SLOW COOKER SIZE:
6 to 7 quart (6 to 7 L)

YIELD: 12 to 14 servings

Crustless Pumpkin Pie

If you're anything like me, you eat the pumpkin pie filling, but you could take or leave the crust. The pumpkin pie filling is where it's at, and this crustless pumpkin pie won't disappoint. I've made this into a healthier version without losing any of the deliciousness of traditional pumpkin pie. It's creamy and scrumptious!

1 can (15 ounces, or 425 g) pumpkin purée
½ cup (115 g) nonfat plain Greek yogurt
2 eggs
1 tablespoon (14 ml) maple syrup
2 teaspoons (10 ml) vanilla
¼ cup (60 g) brown sugar
1 teaspoon pumpkin pie spice
2 tablespoons (16 g) cornstarch

» Line your crock with parchment paper and spray it with nonstick cooking spray.

» In a bowl, mix together the pumpkin purée, yogurt, eggs, maple syrup, and vanilla. When that is well mixed, stir in the sugar and pumpkin pie spice. Lastly, stir in the cornstarch. Pour the mixture into the crock.

» Cover the crock and cook on LOW for 2½ hours. (I do not suggest cooking this on HIGH.)

RECOMMENDED SLOW COOKER SIZE:
3 quart (3 L)

YIELD: 8 servings

Salted Caramel Swirled Brownies

Brownies are amazing, but brownies with caramel in them are *more* than amazing. Impress your family with these sticky, gooey, delicious brownies.

1 box (22 ounces, or 625 g) chocolate
   cake mix
1 cup (235 ml) evaporated milk
4 tablespoons (55 g) butter, melted
¼ cup (50 g) coconut oil, melted
1 cup (235 ml) Caramel Sauce (page 165)
¾ teaspoon sea salt

» Line your crock with a large sheet of parchment paper and spray it with nonstick cooking spray.

» In a bowl, mix together the cake mix, evaporated milk, butter, and oil. Spread half of the batter into the bottom of your crock.

» Pour the Caramel Sauce on top of the brownie batter and sprinkle it with the salt. Finish by spooning the remaining brownie batter on top of the caramel. Using a knife, swirl the caramel and brownie mix.

» Cover the crock and cook on LOW for 6 to 7 hours, or until the brownie is set in the middle. (I do not recommend cooking this on HIGH.)

RECOMMENDED SLOW COOKER SIZE:
6 quart (6 L) or larger

YIELD: 8 to 10 servings

TIPS & SUGGESTIONS

» When removing these easily from the crock pot, lift the parchment paper off carefully first.
» Let these cool completely on a wire rack before cutting and serving.

DREAMY DESSERTS

Irish Cream Brownies

If you're a fan of Irish cream liqueur, then you'll definitely be a fan of these decadent brownies. You'll have a hard time deciding whether you'll want to share these little powder sugar dusted gems.

⅔ cup (85 g) gluten-free flour,
   such as Cup4Cup

⅔ cup (120 g) granulated sugar

⅓ cup (25 g) cocoa powder

¼ teaspoon salt

⅔ cup (155 ml) Irish cream liquor

⅓ cup (80 ml) melted coconut oil

1 egg, lightly beaten

1½ teaspoons vanilla

¼ cup (30 g) or less powdered sugar

» Line your crock with parchment paper and spray it well with nonstick cooking spray.

» In a bowl, mix together the flour, sugar, cocoa powder, and salt.

» In a separate bowl, mix together the liqueur, oil, egg, and vanilla.

» Pour the wet ingredients into the dry ingredients and mix only until all is blended together.

» Pour the batter into the crock and spread it out as evenly as possible.

» Cover the crock and cook on LOW for 2 hours. (I do not recommend cooking this on HIGH.)

» When they are done, remove the brownies from the crock by pulling on the edges of the parchment paper. When the brownies are completely cooled, dust them with powdered sugar.

RECOMMENDED SLOW COOKER SIZE:
5 to 6 quart (5 to 6 L)

YIELD: 8 to 10 servings

TIPS & SUGGESTIONS

Let these cool completely on a wire rack before cutting and serving.

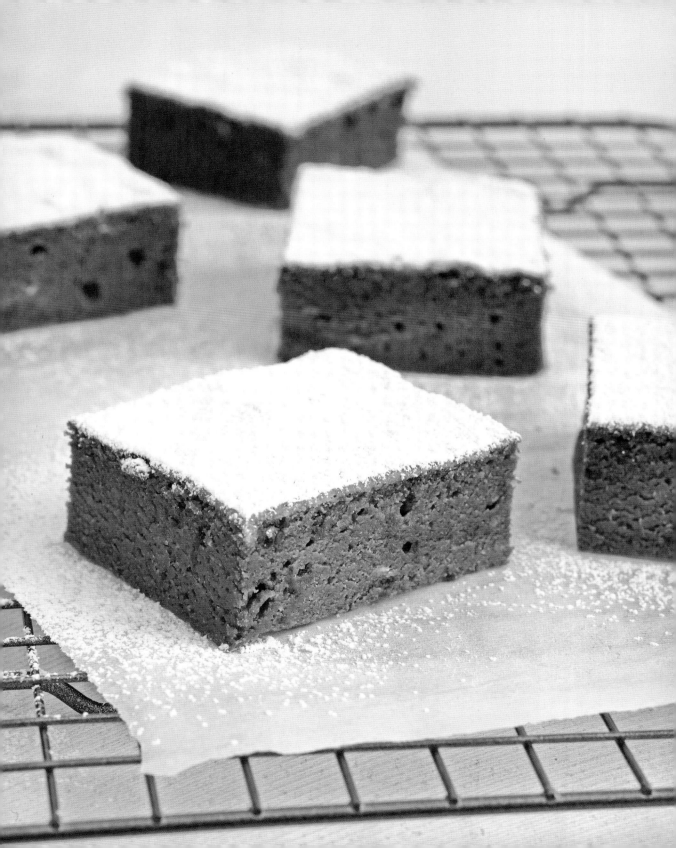

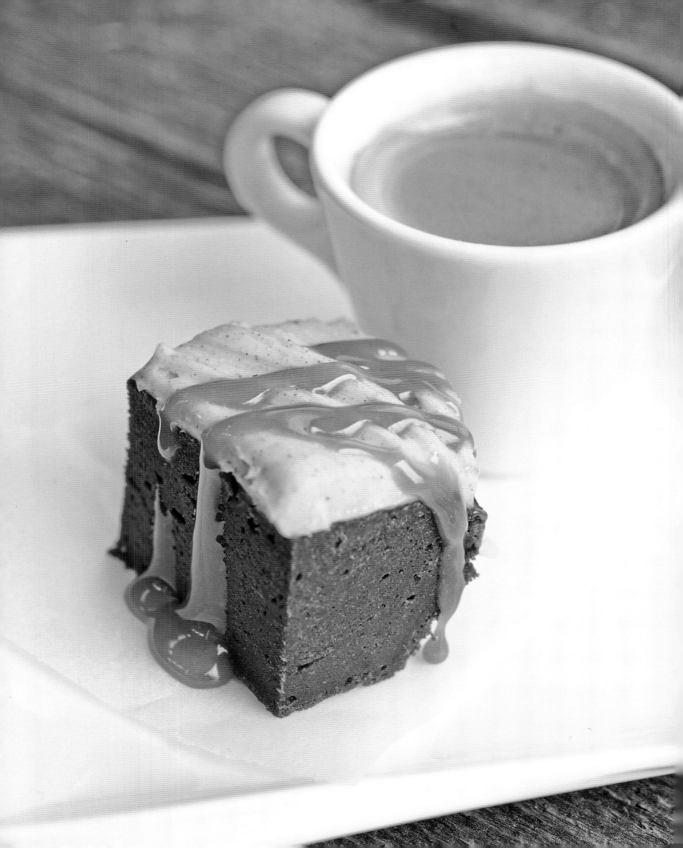

Pumpkin Brownies with Cream Cheese Frosting

5 INGREDIENTS OR LESS

These brownies are the perfect combination of sweet and savory, finished with a homemade just-sweet-enough pumpkin cream cheese frosting. You won't believe how easy these brownies are to make.

FOR THE BROWNIES:

1 box (16 ounces, or 455 g) gluten-free brownie mix

1 can (15 ounce,s or 425 g) pumpkin purée

FOR THE FROSTING:

1 package (8 ounces, or 225 g) reduced fat cream cheese, softened

⅓ cup (40 g) powdered sugar

1 teaspoon pumpkin pie spice

» **To make the brownies:** Line your crock with parchment paper and spray it well with nonstick cooking spray.

» In a bowl, mix the brownie mix with the pumpkin purée. Pour the mixture into the crock and spread it out evenly.

» Cover the crock and cook on LOW for 7 hours or on HIGH for 3½ hours.

» When the brownies are done, remove them from the crock by pulling them out with the parchment paper edges. Place them on a cooling rack.

» **To make the frosting:** When the brownies are just about cool, you can begin working on your frosting. In a bowl, mix together the cream cheese, sugar, and pumpkin pie spice. Spread it over the top of your brownies.

RECOMMENDED SLOW COOKER SIZE:
5 to 6 quart (5 to 6 L)

YIELD: 10 to 15 servings

TIPS & SUGGESTIONS

» Keep these refrigerated if using the cream cheese frosting.

» Top with Caramel Sauce, page 165, if desired.

Apple Berry Crisp

Blueberries, strawberries, and apples with a homemade "crisp" topping make this dessert absolutely irresistible! Served by itself, over ice cream, or even over a gluten-free sponge cake, it is incredibly delicious and comforting.

FOR THE FILLING:

1½ cups (375 g) sliced apples

1½ cups (230 g) frozen blueberries

2 cups (510 g) frozen strawberries

¼ cup (50 g) turbinado sugar

2 teaspoons (10 ml) fresh squeezed orange juice

1 teaspoon vanilla

1 teaspoon orange zest

¼ cup (30 g) cornstarch

1 teaspoon cinnamon

¼ teaspoon nutmeg

FOR THE TOPPING:

½ cup (100 g) turbinado sugar

2 tablespoons (15 g) cornstarch

½ teaspoon cinnamon

⅛ teaspoon salt

3 tablespoons (45 g) cold unsalted butter, sliced into smaller pieces

¼ cup (25 g) chopped pecans

½ cup (40 g) old-fashioned oats

» To make the filling: Spray your crock with nonstick cooking spray. Place the apples, blueberries, and strawberries into the crock. Add in the sugar, orange juice, vanilla, orange zest, cornstarch, cinnamon, and nutmeg. Stir it up.

» To make the topping: In a bowl, mix together the sugar, cornstarch, cinnamon, and salt. Place the butter slices on top. Using a pastry cutter or two forks, cut the butter into the mixture until it is crumbly. Once it's crumbly, gently stir in the pecans and oats. Pour the mixture over the top of the berry mixture.

» Cover the crock and cook on LOW for 4 hours or on HIGH for 2 hours.

RECOMMENDED SLOW COOKER SIZE:
2 to 3 quart (2 to 3 L)

YIELD: 8 to 10 servings

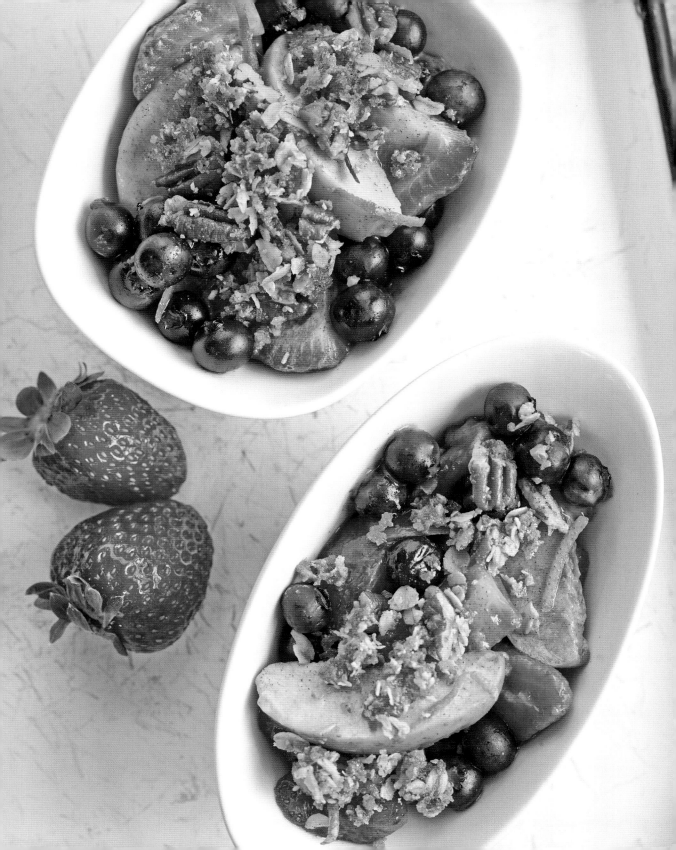

Peach Cobbler

 DAIRY-FREE

There's nothing better than warm, sweet, juicy peaches over a perfectly spongy layer of soft biscuit. Although this recipe doesn't qualify as "5 ingredients or less," it's still super simple at only six ingredients. It's simple, sweet, and incredibly satisfying.

1 cup (125 g) gluten-free baking mix, such as Bisquick

½ teaspoon cinnamon

1 cup (235 ml) almond milk

1 cup (200 g) coconut oil, melted

3 cups (510 g) fresh sliced peaches

1 cup (200 g) turbinado sugar

» Spray your crock with nonstick cooking spray.

» In a bowl, mix together the baking mix, cinnamon, milk, and oil. Pour the mixture into the crock.

» In a bowl, mix together the peaches and sugar. Pour the peaches on top of the batter already in the crock.

» Cover the crock and cook on LOW for 3 hours or on HIGH for 1½ hours.

RECOMMENDED SLOW COOKER SIZE:
2 to 3 quart (2 to 3 L)

YIELD: 6 to 8 servings

Apple Cinnamon Spice Cobbler

"Gooey goodness" is the best way I can describe this delicious recipe. With a cake mix, a few simple spices, and some apples, you have a delicious, moist dessert.

1 box (22 ounces, or 625 g) gluten-free yellow cake mix

1 teaspoon cinnamon

½ teaspoon nutmeg

¼ teaspoon ginger

¼ teaspoon ground cloves

½ cup (115 g) brown sugar

4 fuji, gala, or honeycrisp apples, peeled and sliced

4 tablespoons (55 g) butter, melted

» Line your crock with a sheet of parchment paper and spray it with nonstick cooking spray.

» In a bowl, mix together the cake mix, cinnamon, nutmeg, ginger, cloves, and sugar.

» Put the apple slices into the bowl and pour the butter over the top. Mix it well then pour all the contents into the crock.

» Cover the crock and cook on LOW for 7 to 8 hours or on HIGH for 3½ to 4 hours.

RECOMMENDED SLOW COOKER SIZE:
5 quart (5 L) or larger

YIELD: 8 to 10 servings

 TIPS & SUGGESTIONS

These recipes are absolutely fantastic on their own, but even more delicious served with some vanilla ice cream or frozen yogurt.

Apple Butter

 DAIRY-FREE

Apple butter is delicious on so many things. You can spread it on rice cakes, bread, or crackers or you can mix some into your applesauce or yogurt. This apple butter will not disappoint the masses! Freeze it, put it in a mason jar and tie a cute ribbon around it for a gift, or eat it up right away.

6 pounds (2.7 kg) apples, such as fuji, gala, or honeycrisp

½ cup (115 g) brown sugar

1 cup (200 g) turbinado sugar

1 cup (235 ml) lemon juice

1 teaspoon vanilla

2 tablespoons (14 g) cinnamon

1 teaspoon ground cloves

½ teaspoon nutmeg

Pinch of salt

» Spray your crock with nonstick cooking spray.

» Place all of the ingredients into the crock and mix them up well.

» Cover the crock and cook on LOW for 12 hours. (I do not recommend cooking this on HIGH.)

» Using an immersion blender, purée the apple butter until it's nice and smooth. (If the apple butter is not as thick as you would like it, let it continue to cook for 2 more hours with the lid off of the slow cooker.)

» Store the apple butter in the refrigerator for up to 2 weeks or in the freezer for around 2 months.

RECOMMENDED SLOW COOKER SIZE:
6 quart (6 L) or larger

YIELD: 18 to 24 cups

 ## TIPS & SUGGESTIONS

» If you don't have an immersion blender, you can use a food processor, or even a blender, to purée the apple butter in small batches.

» If you're using a blender, be sure to cover the top with a towel. It would not be good for hot liquid to spray all over you and your kitchen!

» If you're a canner, can this apple butter. It would be wonderful to be able to pull it out of the pantry year round. It would also make a lovely gift!

DREAMY DESSERTS

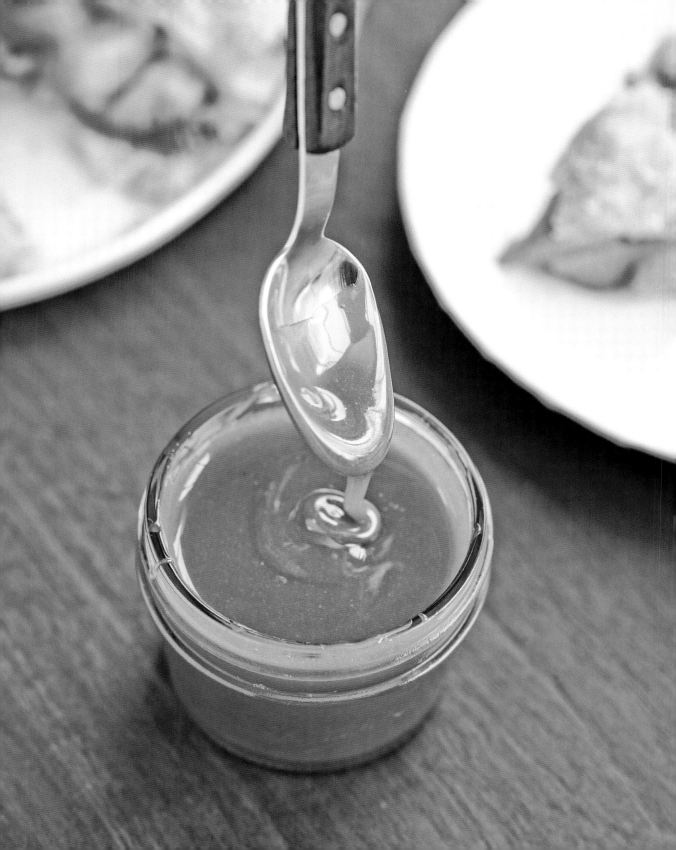

Caramel Sauce

 INGREDIENTS OR LESS

Are you ready to make the easiest and most delicious caramel ever? This caramel turns out absolutely perfectly in the slow cooker. It has just the perfect amount of sweetness, a beautiful rich color, and a nice smooth texture. You'll never buy store-bought caramel again!

4 cans (each 14 ounces, or 395 g) sweetened condensed milk

6 mason jars (6 ounces, or 175 ml, each)

» Pour the condensed milk evenly into the mason jars. Close them tightly and place them into your crock.

» Add water to your crock until the milk is covered. The jar does not need to be covered.

» Cover the crock and cook on LOW for 8 hours. Carefully remove the jars and let them cool on the counter. (I do not recommend cooking this on HIGH.)

RECOMMENDED SLOW COOKER SIZE:
5 quart (5 L) or larger

YIELD: 6 mason jars (6 ounces, or 175 ml, each)

 ## TIPS & SUGGESTIONS

» These will last unopened for 1 month, or opened for 1 week. Refrigeration is suggested.

» To warm the caramel, simply place the jar in the microwave without the lid on and microwave for about 30 seconds at a time until the caramel reaches your desired consistency.

» The longer you cook this, the thicker the caramel becomes.

Strawberry Orange Sauce

 DAIRY-FREE

"Pure deliciousness" is how I describe this sauce. It's smooth and decadent, and the combination of the strawberries and orange juice create a perfect marriage of flavors. Delight your palette with this tantalizing sauce!

2 cups (510 g) frozen strawberries

½ cup (115 g) brown sugar

2 tablespoons (28 ml) fresh squeezed orange juice

1 teaspoon orange zest

½ teaspoon cinnamon

2 tablespoons (16 g) cornstarch

» Spray your crock with nonstick cooking spray.

» Place the strawberries into the crock and add in the remaining ingredients. Stir it around.

» Cover the crock and cook on LOW for 4 to 4½ hours. (I do not recommend cooking this on HIGH.)

» When the cook time is up, using an immersion blender, purée the sauce until it's smooth.

RECOMMENDED SLOW COOKER SIZE:
1 quart (1 L)

YIELD: 15 to 18 servings

 ## TIPS & SUGGESTIONS

» **This sauce is amazing over vanilla ice cream or frozen yogurt.**

» **You can also drizzle the sauce into some plain yogurt or even over the top of a cheesecake.**

» **If you chill this sauce, it is excellent spread on some gluten-free toast or a gluten-free bagel with cream cheese.**

ACKNOWLEDGMENTS

I am truly blessed to have an amazing support network of family and friends. Life has brought me many surprises along the way. Many of my dreams have come true, and some are yet to be. Publishing this book is definitely a dream come true. God blessed me with many gifts, including the ability to share my love for cooking, developing recipes, and writing about them in a way that touches people. There is not a day that goes by when I am not truly thankful for these gifts.

This book would not have been possible without the help of many, many people.

To my incredible husband, Justin: You cheered me on every single day, cooked, cleaned, washed slow cookers, ran errands, did laundry, kept the kids busy, high-fived me, encouraged me, celebrated with me, and lifted me up when I was down. I don't think I could ever repay you for all you've done. I love you more than words can say.

To my daughter, Ella: My sweet, positive, cheerful little girl who never once complained while Mommy worked on her cookbook. You are my sunshine. You make me smile. Thank you for eating all of my recipes and for always finding a positive way to be truthful with me. I am proud of you—every single day.

To my son, Gavin: My giggly, fun, and silly little boy who worked beside me in the kitchen, wanting to help me with each new recipe. Thank you for being my right-hand man in the kitchen. I hope we cook together for more years to come. You are my happy little guy who can always make Mommy laugh. I couldn't have asked for a more loving little boy.

To my amazing family: You never stopped encouraging me and telling me how proud you are of me. I can't express to you how much that has meant to me. I love you all.

To all my friends: Thank you to those who gave me ideas, offered me advice, tasted my recipes, and gave me endless encouragement. Maria Shevlin, many special thanks to you for testing recipes for me, and letting me bounce ideas off you day after day. You are an amazing friend, and I am forever grateful to have you in my life.

To all my blog followers and readers: I want to thank all of you for your understanding, loyalty, and patience. This book would not have been possible without you. Thank you for reading my blog, cooking my recipes, and sharing them with your family and friends.

ABOUT THE AUTHOR

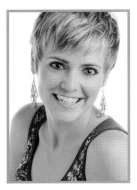

Hope Comerford is a mom, wife, elementary/music teacher, blogger, recipe developer, public speaker, FitAddict Training fit leader, Young Living Essential Oils enthusiast/teacher, and published author. In 2013, she was diagnosed with gluten intolerance, and since then she has spent many hours creating easy, practical, and delicious gluten-free recipe that can be enjoyed by people who are affected by gluten and those who are not.

Growing up, Hope spent many hours in the kitchen with her Meme (grandmother), and her love for cooking grew from there. While working on her master's degree when her daughter was young, Hope turned to her slow cookers for some salvation and sanity. It was from there she began truly experimenting with recipes and quickly learned she had the ability to get a little more creative in the kitchen and develop her own recipes. She started her blog, A Busy Mom's Slow Cooker Adventures located at www.slowcookeradventures.com in 2010 to simply share the recipes she was making with her family and friends. She never imagined people all over the world would begin visiting her page and sharing her recipes with others as well. In 2013, Hope self-published her first cookbook *Slow Cooker Recipes 10 Ingredients or Less and Gluten-Free*. It was one of the proudest moments of her life.

Hope lives in the city of Clinton Township, Michigan, near Metro Detroit. She's been a native of Michigan her whole life. She has been happily married to her husband and best friend, Justin, for nine years. Together they have two children, Ella (age 7) and Gavin (age 4).

You can follow Hope on all of the following social media outlets and reach her at:

www.slowcookeradventures.com

Facebook: www.fb.com/SlowCookerAdventures

Twitter: @BusyCrockPotMom

Pinterest: pinterest.com/BusyCrockPotMom

Instagram: SlowCookerAdventures

YouTube: www.youtube.com/slowcookeradventures

Email: hope@slowcookeradventures.com

INDEX